Clinical Manual of
Anxiety Disorders

Clinical Manual of Anxiety Disorders

Edited by

Dan J. Stein, M.D., Ph.D.

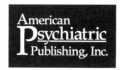

American Psychiatric Publishing, Inc.

Washington, DC
London, England

Copyright © 2004 American Psychiatric Publishing, Inc.
ALL RIGHTS RESERVED

Diagnostic criteria included in this book are reprinted, with permission, from *Diagnostic and Statistical Manual of Mental Disorders,* 4th Edition, Text Revision. Copyright © 2000, American Psychiatric Association.

Manufactured in the United States of America on acid-free paper
07   06   05   04   5   4   3   2   1
First Edition

Typeset in Adobe's Garamond and Formata

American Psychiatric Publishing, Inc.
1000 Wilson Boulevard
Arlington, VA 22209-3901
www.appi.org

Library of Congress Cataloging-in-Publication Data

Clinical manual of anxiety disorders / edited by Dan J. Stein.—1st ed.
        p. ; cm
Includes bibliographical references and index.
    ISBN 1-58562-076-9 (alk. paper)
  1. Anxiety—Handbooks, manuals, etc. 2. Anxiety—Treatment—Handbooks, manuals, etc.
    [DNLM: 1. Anxiety Disorders—diagnosis. 2. Anxiety disorders—therapy. WM 172 C64183 2004] I. Stein, Dan J.
    RC531.C585 2004
    616.85′22—dc22

                                                            2003058259

British Library Cataloguing in Publication Data
A CIP record is available from the British Library.

Contents

4 Social Phobia 63

Franklin R. Schneier, M.D.
Jane A. Luterek, M.A.
Richard G. Heimberg, Ph.D.
Eduardo Leonardo, M.D., Ph.D.

Contributors

Richard G. Heimberg, Ph.D.
Professor of Psychology; Director, Clinical Psychology Training Program; and Director, Adult Anxiety Clinic of Temple, Department of Psychology, Temple University, Philadelphia, Pennsylvania

Jonathan D. Huppert, Ph.D.
Assistant Professor of Psychology in Psychiatry, Center for the Treatment and Study of Anxiety, University of Pennsylvania, Philadelphia, Pennsylvania

Michael Jenike, M.D.
Professor of Psychiatry and Director, OCD Clinic and Neuroscience Program, Massachusetts General Hospital, Harvard Medical School, Charlestown, Massachusetts

Nancy J. Keuthen, Ph.D.
Chief Psychologist, OCD Clinic, Massachusetts General Hospital, Charlestown, Massachusetts

Gustavo Kinrys, M.D.
Anxiety Disorders Program, Massachusetts General Hospital; Assistant Professor of Psychiatry, Department of Psychiatry, Harvard Medical School, Boston, Massachusetts

Eduardo Leonardo, M.D., Ph.D.
Postdoctoral Clinical Fellow in Psychiatry, New York State Psychiatric Institute, Columbia University College of Physicians and Surgeons, New York, New York

Jane A. Luterek, M.A.
Department of Psychology, Temple University, Philadelphia, Pennsylvania

Randall D. Marshall, M.D.
Director of Trauma Studies and Services, New York State Psychiatric Institute; Associate Professor of Clinical Psychiatry, Columbia University College of Physicians and Surgeons, New York, New York

Brian Martis, M.D.
Clinical Assistant Professor, Trauma Stress and Anxiety Research Center/University of Michigan Depression Center, Department of Psychiatry, Ann Arbor, Michigan

Mark H. Pollack, M.D.
Director, Anxiety Disorders Program, Massachusetts General Hospital; Associate Professor of Psychiatry, Harvard Medical School, Boston, Massachusetts

Barbara Rothbaum, Ph.D.
Director, Trauma and Anxiety Recovery Program, and Associate Professor in Psychiatry, Emory University School of Medicine, Atlanta, Georgia

Moira Rynn, M.D.
Assistant Professor of Psychiatry and Medical Director, Mood and Anxiety Disorders Section, Department of Psychiatry, University of Pennsylvania, Philadelphia, Pennsylvania

Franklin R. Schneier, M.D.
Research Psychiatrist, Anxiety Disorders Clinic, New York State Psychiatric Institute; Associate Professor of Clinical Psychiatry, Columbia University College of Physicians and Surgeons, New York, New York

Dan J. Stein, M.D., Ph.D.
Director, MRC Unit on Anxiety Disorders, Department of Psychiatry, University of Stellenbosch, Cape Town, South Africa, and University of Florida, Gainesville, Florida

Bavanisha Vythilingum, M.B.
Research Clinician, MRC Unit on Anxiety Disorders, Department of Psychiatry, University of Stellenbosch, Cape Town, South Africa

Kimberly A. Wilson, Ph.D.
Department of Psychiatry and Behavioral Sciences, Stanford University Medical Center, Stanford, California

1

Introduction

Dan J. Stein, M.D., Ph.D.

Concepts of anxiety have long held a central position in philosophical and psychoanalytic theories. Empirical research on anxiety disorders, however, has a relatively short history. Nevertheless, a range of important advances has been made, with significant implications for practicing clinicians. This introductory chapter reviews some of the important diagnostic, epidemiological, neurobiological, and treatment findings; this serves as background to subsequent chapters on each of the individual anxiety disorders.

Diagnosis

In DSM-II (American Psychiatric Association 1968), anxiety disorders fell under the broad umbrella category of "anxiety neurosis." In DSM-III (American Psychiatric Association 1980), the anxiety disorders were separated into a number of discrete conditions, including panic disorder, obsessive-compulsive disorder (OCD), and agoraphobia and other phobias, although generalized anxiety disorder was seen as a residual diagnosis and social phobia could not be diagnosed in the presence of avoidant personality disorder. By DSM-IV-TR (American Psychiatric Association 2000), there was further consolidation of the specificity of each anxiety disorder; generalized anxiety disorder and social phobia were conceptualized as independent entities, and anxiety disorder secondary to substance use and general medical disorders were also defined.

An approach that "splits" the different anxiety disorders offers a number of important potential advantages. Specific diagnoses can be made with a great deal of reliability, then subjected to careful and rigorous research. Such research is potentially able to establish the validity of different diagnoses—demonstrating that a specific diagnosis is useful in terms of predicting clinical features, such as course, and is associated with specific psychobiological mediating factors. Such an approach then lays the way for developing and researching specific interventions for the management of each particular anxiety disorder.

Nevertheless, a "lumper" might point out that splitting the anxiety disorders has a number of potential disadvantages. First, there is significant comorbidity between the different anxiety disorders, as well as with mood disorders, so that this approach may seem artificial. Similarly, important psychobiological features appear to overlap between different anxiety symptoms, suggesting that nature cannot be artificially carved at the joints. Even from the point of view of treatment, psychotherapeutic and pharmacotherapeutic principles often overlap across the different anxiety disorders.

To some extent, the optimal approach used may depend on the setting. In a research setting, it may be important to split as much as possible. DSM-IV-TR offers a number of subtype specifiers, and research instruments allow for various other subtypes to be defined. Such precision may be crucial for further advances in the field. In a primary care setting, however, it is important to put the issue of "anxiety" on the clinicians' radar. If clinicians are aware of a problem—either of anxiety or of avoidance—they can begin with a broad approach, then refer patients on for more specialized assessment and treatment when necessary.

Certainly, it is crucial to be aware of anxiety disorder diagnoses in a range of settings. Anxiety symptoms and disorders in different age groups (from children through to the elderly), in different medical settings (including substance use disorder programs), and in different social and cultural settings are important for the clinician to be aware of. There is increasing use of anxiety disorder screening days to raise awareness of anxiety disorders in the community. Early awareness may ultimately result in better prognosis, with prevention or reduction of comorbid mood disorders so often seen in patients with anxiety disorder.

Anxiety (in some ways the "positive" dimension of anxiety disorders) and avoidance (in some ways their "negative" dimension) are both present in a range of different anxiety disorders. Chapters in this book provide sufficient detail to allow differential diagnosis among the anxiety disorders, as well as differentiation of specific anxiety disorders from other relevant psychiatric and general medical conditions. Each of the chapters also briefly discusses principles of assessment, as well as relevant rating scales that are increasingly used in everyday clinical practice to quantify severity of symptoms and their change over time.

Epidemiology

The development of criteria for specific anxiety disorders has allowed large-scale epidemiological studies of the anxiety disorders in nationally representative and cross-national community settings. Importantly, the anxiety disorders have been shown to be common, chronic, disabling, and costly in both the developed and the developing world. Nevertheless, they are often underdiagnosed and undertreated, and this further contributes to suffering and cost associated with them.

The Epidemiologic Catchment Area (ECA) study was important insofar as it provided evidence that the anxiety disorders comprised the most prevalent group of psychiatric disorders in the United States (Robins et al. 1984). Specific phobia in particular was the most common psychiatric disorder, and OCD was the fourth most common. Anxiety disorders were found to be more common in women. A cross-national study that used a similar methodology yielded similar findings in a range of different countries (Weissman et al. 1997).

The National Comorbidity Survey (NCS) employed updated diagnostic criteria and again demonstrated that the anxiety disorders were the most prevalent group of psychiatric disorders in the United States (Kessler et al. 1994). Social phobia in particular was found to be a highly prevalent disorder in the community. This survey did not, however, address OCD. Furthermore, neither the ECA study nor the NCS included obsessive-compulsive spectrum disorders in the diagnostic instrument, despite data suggesting these conditions also have a high prevalence.

Clinical studies have confirmed the high prevalence of the anxiety disorders. In primary care clinics, the most common anxiety disorder is generalized anxiety disorder, a condition that may be associated with particularly high medical system use (Kessler 2000). There may also be other interesting differences between clinical and community samples; for example, although social phobia is more common in women in the community, men appear to be more likely to seek clinical treatment.

In both the ECA study and the NCS, anxiety disorders were found to often have early onset and precede the development of other disorders (particularly mood disorders). One-year prevalence was often similar to lifetime prevalence, suggesting that these disorders have a chronic course. More clinical studies, such as the Harvard/Brown Anxiety Disorders Program (Yonkers et al. 2000), have confirmed that anxiety disorders often have onset in childhood or adolescence and are characterized by significant comorbidity and chronicity.

There is growing appreciation of the extent to which anxiety disorders are accompanied by objective disability and subjectively impaired quality of life (Mogotsi et al. 2000). Of course, distress and dysfunction are, by DSM-IV-TR definition, necessary for the distinction between symptoms and disorder. However, recent data have provided insight into the severity and range of impairments in anxiety disorders. For example, in one important study, OCD was found to be the tenth most disabling of all medical disorders (Murray and Lopez 1996). These disorders affect function in academic and occupational settings and negatively affect relationships with family and friends. Furthermore, given their early onset, anxiety disorders may adversely affect normal developmental processes.

The financial cost of anxiety disorders has also been increasingly documented. An early set of data suggested that anxiety disorders accounted for one-third of the costs of psychiatric disorders (Dupont et al. 1996). This amounts to several billions of dollars each year. These costs are primarily indirect (i.e., affecting occupational and social functioning) rather than direct (i.e., affecting cost of medical treatment). Subsequent surveys have consolidated these findings (Greenberg et al. 1999). Early diagnosis and rigorous treatment of the anxiety disorders may well prove to be highly cost-effective.

Pathogenesis

Study of anxiety disorders is made easier by the fact that animal models provide windows into both the proximal and the distal mechanisms involved in mediating these conditions. Study of processes such as fear conditioning, for example, allows an exploration of the neurocircuitry and neurochemicals involved in fear acquisition and desensitization. On the other hand, the study of ethology, as Darwin long ago pointed out, allows one to determine the evolutionary basis of different kinds of anxiety—on the basis of the hypothesis that anxiety serves as a useful survival mechanism (Darwin 1965).

Fear conditioning has been a particularly useful paradigm (Davis and Whalen 2001; Le Doux 1998). The amygdala and its afferents and efferents play a crucial role in fear acquisition and responses (and perhaps in mediating the "positive" anxious symptoms of anxiety disorders). Furthermore, the hippocampus appears to play an important role in remembering the context in which fear conditioning has taken place (and perhaps in mediating the "negative" avoidance symptoms of anxiety disorders). There is some evidence, too, that implicit amygdala-based and explicit hippocampus-based cognitive-affective processes can be dissociated from one another (Bechara et al. 1995).

Various neurochemical systems found in, or affecting, these important neurocircuits likely play an important role in the anxiety disorders. Early work focused on the noradrenergic system in anxiety, but the efficacy of serotonin reuptake inhibitors has also led to a focus on serotonin receptors and subreceptors. Faster-acting excitatory and inhibitory systems, such as glutamate and GABA (γ-aminobutyric acid) neurotransmission, are perhaps equally important in anxiety, as evidenced by the anxiolytic effects of benzodiazepines. Neuroendocrine changes (including hypothalamic-pituitary-adrenal axis dysfunction) and neuroimmunological disruptions may also play a crucial role in some anxiety disorders.

Increasingly, research at a molecular level promises to shed light on the proximal mechanisms underlying anxiety and anxiety disorders. Data are increasing on, for example, the genetics of fear conditioning and the molecular aspects of signal transduction in anxiety disorders. In particular, there is a growing appreciation of the role of second and third messengers and ultimately of genetic transcription and neuronal plasticity in anxiety and mood disorders (Lesch 2001). We can hope that a more complete understanding of the molecular underpinnings of anxiety will lead to novel treatments for patients with anxiety disorders.

It is relevant to emphasize that work on the molecular aspects of anxiety disorders does not create a wall between nature and nurture in our understanding of the pathogenesis of these conditions. On the contrary, we now know that early trauma has an impact on neurocircuitry, neurochemistry, and neuroendocrinology (Sanchez et al. 2001). The precise nature of this mediation requires further exploration, but the amygdala and hippocampus may well be involved. Conversely, we are increasingly aware that both pharmacotherapy and psychotherapy can normalize dysfunctional circuits in anxiety disorders (Baxter et al. 1992; Furmark et al. 2002).

There have also been advances in understanding the distal evolutionary bases for anxiety disorders. Two kinds of general evolutionary approaches to anxiety symptoms are possible; the first emphasizes the role of anxiety as a normal defense that promotes *survival,* whereas the second focuses on the possibility that certain kinds of anxiety represent *defects.* Fever during an infection, for example, is defensive insofar as it serves to help combat the foreign agent. Similarly, social anxiety is particularly useful for a social primate that needs to be aware of social threats, thus accounting for the high prevalence of this phenomenon in humans.

On the other hand, anxiety may in certain instances seem defective. For many years, posttraumatic stress disorder (PTSD) was thought of as a normal reaction to an abnormal event. But we increasingly think of PTSD in terms of an abnormal response, perhaps mediated by particular neurotransmitter and neuroendocrine dysfunctions (Yehuda and McFarlane 1995). Similarly, different anxiety disorders may be characterized by different kinds of "false alarms"; these psychobiological dysfunctions prove to be problematic for those who experience them (Stein and Bouwer 1997).

Management

Early psychotherapeutic intervention for anxiety disorders was based on psychoanalytic principles and relied on theories about the unconscious. In phar macotherapy, the development of the benzodiazepines was a substantial advance beyond earlier use of more dangerous pharmacological agents. Recent decades have seen the introduction of evidence-based psychotherapies and the development of more effective and better-tolerated pharmacological agents for the treatment of anxiety disorders. In the past few years, the first medications have also been registered for the treatment of previously neglected disorders such as social phobia.

Evidence-based psychotherapy for anxiety disorders primarily comprises behavioral and cognitive interventions. These interventions, which emphasize principles of exposure, hierarchical desensitization, and cognitive restructuring, are perhaps particularly important to consider when avoidance symptoms dominate the clinical picture. Although the efficacy of these interventions has been demonstrated in a range of randomized controlled trials, experienced cognitive-behavioral psychotherapists are not available in all settings, and additional work is needed to educate clinicians in their optimal use. Furthermore, there is a need for more work to determine the active ingredients that underlie the efficacy of cognitive-behavioral interventions.

Benzodiazepines continue to play a role in short-term treatment of anxiety symptoms, but selective serotonin reuptake inhibitors (SSRIs) have become a first-line treatment for a range of different anxiety disorders. Benzodiazepines have a number of significant disadvantages, including cognitive impairment, relative contraindication during exposure therapies, and problems on withdrawal. SSRIs, in contrast, are both effective and reasonably well tolerated, and an added advantage is that they are useful for both anxiety symptoms and comorbid mood disorders. More recently introduced medications, such as the serotonergic-noradrenergic reuptake inhibitors and the noradrenergic reuptake inhibitors, may also have useful roles.

There is a relative lack of long-term data on the pharmacotherapy and psychotherapy of anxiety disorders. Given the chronicity of anxiety disorders, this is an important gap. Nevertheless, a number of lessons are apparent. First, early tapering of medication often leads to relapse. Second, medications that are useful in the acute phase typically retain efficacy and tolerability when used over the longer term. Thus, expert consensus reviews have by and large recommended that medication for anxiety disorders be continued for 1–2 years. Third, psychotherapy may be particularly helpful in maintenance of treatment response, although additional work is needed to provide unequivocal data.

Other areas in which more research is required are the treatment of anxiety disorders in younger and older patients, in patients with comorbid disorders including substance use disorders, and in primary care settings. Indeed, though randomized controlled trials have often demonstrated efficacy, there is less work demonstrating effectiveness in naturalistic treatment settings, where a broader range of patients with anxiety disorder is seen, including patients with increased comorbidity. More research on the optimal combination and sequencing of pharmacotherapy and psychotherapy would also be helpful. In the interim, however, it seems reasonable to use a combination of antidepressants and cognitive-behavioral principles for many patients with anxiety disorders.

Many of these patients respond to first-line interventions, but the subgroup of nonresponders is an important one. There is a relative lack of controlled augmentation studies in the management of refractory anxiety disorders, but even here there has been progress. Thus, for example, in OCD, there is now good evidence that augmentation of SRIs with low-dose dopamine blockers is useful (McDougle et al. 2000). Furthermore, a number of novel interventions for treatment-refractory anxiety disorders are under development, including transcranial magnetic stimulation and deep brain stimulation. Pharmacological prophylaxis against disorders such as PTSD is also being investigated (Pitman et al. 2002).

A range of interventions other than traditional pharmacotherapy and individual psychotherapy may also be important in optimizing management of anxiety disorders. Simply providing education (psychoeducation) may play a crucial role in dispelling myths and in encouraging people to view anxiety disorders as medical conditions that can be diagnosed and treated. Formal introduction of evidence-based guidelines and algorithms into health care systems may have a role in improving treatments. Media campaigns and direct-to-consumer marketing, bibliotherapy and Internet support, consumer advocacy, and family interventions may all have a role in increasing awareness of anxiety disorders, in encouraging early diagnosis and treatment, and in facilitating adherence to appropriate treatment (Stein 1997; Stein et al. 2001).

To conclude, it may be useful to summarize some of the general principles of management across different anxiety disorders (Table 1–1). First, a thorough psychiatric and medical history and examination should allow for a DSM-IV-TR diagnosis, assessment of comorbid disorders, and the exclusion of underlying general medical disorders that might account for the anxiety

Table 1–1.   Treatment principles in anxiety disorders

- Determine DSM-IV-TR diagnosis (requires thorough psychiatric history and examination)

- Rule out underlying general medical disorders (requires medical history and examination)

- Assess comorbidity, impairment, and symptom severity (standardized rating scales may be helpful)

- Understand the patient's explanatory model, share information, negotiate a shared model and treatment plan

- Consider including family members in the treatment plan (particularly if they are facilitating avoidance)

- Consider selective serotonin reuptake inhibitor: start low (particularly in panic) and end high (particularly in obsessive-compulsive disorder), for a trial of 10–12 weeks, with maintenance lasting at least 1 year

- Encourage self-monitoring, countering of catastrophic thoughts, increased exposure, and decreased avoidance

symptoms at hand. Although this will also provide information about symptom severity and associated disability, standardized rating scales are useful for rigorously assessing the clinical picture and monitoring change. A crucial next step is to understand patients' own explanatory model of their symptoms and to provide information about current psychiatric models so that a shared understanding and treatment plan can be negotiated. In some cases, the family may also need to be involved in this negotiation (for example, in cases in which family members facilitate avoidant behavior).

This plan may at times focus on pharmacotherapy or psychotherapy, but in many cases both modalities will be used. SSRIs, for example, have consistently been shown to be effective in almost all anxiety disorders and are also useful for comorbid depression. A general principle would be to start at low doses (particularly in patients with panic attacks), but for a trial period to last 10–12 weeks and to end at high doses if necessary (perhaps particularly in OCD). Short-term addition of benzodiazepines to an antidepressant may be considered in cases in which rapid symptom relief is crucial. At the same time, basic techniques of cognitive-behavioral therapy are useful alone or in combination with medication: self-monitoring to increase awareness, countering of catastrophic thoughts, and increasing exposure to and decreasing avoidance of anxiety-provoking stimuli. Medication should be continued well beyond the acute phase, but it is possible that cognitive-behavioral therapy techniques are useful in preventing relapse once medication is gradually tapered.

General principles of this kind can be followed in primary care settings. In more specialized settings, it is possible to make particular modifications for each individual anxiety disorder to optimize outcome. For this reason, patients whose condition fails to respond to an adequate trial of medication or cognitive-behavioral psychotherapy given in a primary care setting should be referred to a specialist. Details of the management of specific anxiety disorders are discussed in the remaining chapters.

Conclusion

Anxiety disorders are among the most prevalent, persistent, disabling, and costly of psychiatric disorders. The fact that they remain underdiagnosed and undertreated deserves attention. Animal models provide an important basis for future psychobiological research, and we can look forward to future delineation of the genetic and molecular bases of anxiety disorders. Treatment of anxiety disorders is increasingly evidence based, and there is a rationale for combining certain pharmacotherapies (e.g., serotonergic antidepressants) with certain psychotherapy principles (e.g., encouraging exposure). Additional effectiveness studies and long-term studies are needed, but in the interim, we can approach the treatment of anxiety disorder patients with confidence, in the expectation that current tools for assessment and intervention will very often lead to successful outcomes. I hope that clinicians find this volume useful in obtaining such results.

References

American Psychiatric Association: Diagnostic and Statistical Manual of Mental Disorders, 2nd Edition. Washington, DC, American Psychiatric Association, 1968

American Psychiatric Association: Diagnostic and Statistical Manual of Mental Disorders, 3rd Edition. Washington, DC, American Psychiatric Association, 1980

American Psychiatric Association: Diagnostic and Statistical Manual of Mental Disorders, 4th Edition, Text Revision. Washington, DC, American Psychiatric Association, 2000

Baxter LR, Schwartz JM, Bergman KS, et al: Caudate glucose metabolic rate changes with both drug and behavior therapy for OCD. Arch Gen Psychiatry 49:681–689, 1992

Bechara A, Tranel D, Damasio H, et al: Double dissociation of conditioning and declarative knowledge relative to the amygdala and hippocampus in humans. Science 269:1115–1118, 1995

Darwin C: The Expression of Emotion in Man and Animals (1872). Chicago, IL, University of Chicago Press, 1965

Davis M, Whalen PJ: The amygdala: vigilance and emotion. Mol Psychiatry 6:13–34, 2001

Dupont RL, Rice DP, Miller LS, et al: Economic costs of anxiety disorders. Anxiety 2:167–172, 1996

Furmark T, Tillfors M, Marteinsdottir I, et al: Common changes in cerebral blood flow in patients with social phobia treated with citalopram or cognitive-behavioral therapy. Arch Gen Psychiatry 59:425–433, 2002

Greenberg PE, Sisitsky T, Kessler RC, et al: The economic burden of the anxiety disorders in the 1990s. J Clin Psychiatry 60:427–435, 1999

Kessler RC: The epidemiology of pure and comorbid generalized anxiety disorder: a review and evaluation of recent research. Acta Psychiatr Scand Suppl 1 406:7–13, 2000

Kessler RC, McGonagle KC, Zhao S, et al: Lifetime and 12-month prevalence of DSM-III-R psychiatric disorders in the United States: results from the National Comorbidity Survey. Arch Gen Psychiatry 51:8–19, 1994

LeDoux J: Fear and the brain: where have we been, and where are we going? Biol Psychiatry 44:1229–1238, 1998

Lesch KP: Serotonergic gene expression and depression: implications for developing novel antidepressants. J Affect Disord 62:57–76, 2001

McDougle CJ, Epperson CN, Pelton GH, et al: A double-blind, placebo-controlled study of risperidone addition in serotonin reuptake inhibitor-refractory obsessive-compulsive disorder. Arch Gen Psychiatry 57:794–802, 2000

Mogotsi M, Kaminer D, Stein DJ: Quality of life in the anxiety disorders. Harv Rev Psychiatry 8:273–282, 2000

Murray CJL, Lopez AD: Global Burden of Disease: A Comprehensive Assessment of Mortality and Morbidity from Diseases, Injuries, and Risk Factors in 1990 and Projected to 2020, Vol 1. Cambridge, MA, Harvard University Press, 1996

Pitman RK, Sanders KM, Zusman RM, et al: Pilot study of secondary prevention of posttraumatic stress disorder with propranolol. Biol Psychiatry 51:189–192, 2002

Robins LN, Holzer JE, Weissman MM, et al: Lifetime prevalence of specific psychiatric disorders in three sites. Arch Gen Psychiatry 41:949–958, 1984

Sanchez MM, Ladd CO, Plotsky PM: Early adverse experience as a developmental risk factor for later psychopathology: evidence from rodent and primate models. Dev Psychopathol 13:419–449, 2001

Stein DJ: Psychiatry on the Internet: survey of an OCD mailing list. Psychiatr Bull 21:95–98, 1997

Stein DJ, Bouwer C: A neuro-evolutionary approach to the anxiety disorders. J Anxiety Disord 11:409–429, 1997

Stein DJ, Wessels C, Zungu-Dirwayi N, et al: Value and effectiveness of consumer advocacy groups: a survey of the anxiety disorders support group in South Africa. Depress Anxiety 13:105–107, 2001

Weissman MM, Bland RC, Canino GJ, et al: The cross-national epidemiology of panic disorder. Arch Gen Psychiatry 54:305–309, 1997

Yehuda R, McFarlane AC: Conflict between current knowledge about posttraumatic stress disorder and its original conceptual basis. Am J Psychiatry 152:1705–1713, 1995

Yonkers KA, Dyck IR, Warshaw MKMB: Factors predicting the clinical course of generalised anxiety disorder. Br J Psychiatry 176:544–549, 2000

2

Panic Disorder and Agoraphobia

Gustavo Kinrys, M.D.
Mark H. Pollack, M.D.

Phenomenology

Symptoms

Panic disorder is a common, distressing, and often disabling condition in which patients experience recurrent and unexpected panic attacks followed by at least 1 month of persistent concerns about additional attacks (i.e., anticipatory anxiety), worry about the implications of the attack, or significant changes in behavior (e.g., avoidance) related to the attacks (DSM-IV-TR diagnostic criteria; American Psychiatric Association 2000). To meet diagnostic criteria, the attacks neither can be due to the physiological effects of a substance or a medical condition nor can be better accounted for in conjunction with other psychiatric disorders such as social or specific phobia, posttraumatic stress disorder (PTSD), or separation anxiety disorder (Table 2–1).

Table 2–1.   DSM-IV-TR diagnostic criteria for panic disorder

Diagnostic criteria for 300.01 panic disorder without agoraphobia
A. Both (1) and (2):
    (1) recurrent unexpected panic attacks
    (2) at least one of the attacks has been followed by 1 month (or more) of one (or more) of the following:
        (a) persistent concern about having additional attacks
        (b) worry about the implications of the attack or its consequences (e.g., losing control, having a heart attack, "going crazy")
        (c) a significant change in behavior related to the attacks
B. Absence of agoraphobia.
C. The panic attacks are not due to the direct physiological effects of a substance (e.g., a drug of abuse, a medication) or a general medical condition (e.g., hyperthyroidism).
D. The panic attacks are not better accounted for by another mental disorder, such as social phobia (e.g., occurring on exposure to feared social situations), specific phobia (e.g., on exposure to a specific phobic situation), obsessive-compulsive disorder (e.g., on exposure to dirt in someone with an obsession about contamination), posttraumatic stress disorder (e.g., in response to stimuli associated with a severe stressor), or separation anxiety disorder (e.g., in response to being away from home or close relatives).

Diagnostic criteria for 300.21 panic disorder with agoraphobia
A. Both (1) and (2):
    (1) recurrent unexpected panic attacks
    (2) at least one of the attacks has been followed by 1 month (or more) of one (or more) of the following:
        (a) persistent concern about having additional attacks
        (b) worry about the implications of the attack or its consequences (e.g., losing control, having a heart attack, "going crazy")
        (c) a significant change in behavior related to the attacks
B. The presence of agoraphobia.
C. The panic attacks are not due to the direct physiological effects of a substance (e.g., a drug of abuse, a medication) or a general medical condition (e.g., hyperthyroidism).
D. The panic attacks are not better accounted for by another mental disorder, such as social phobia (e.g., occurring on exposure to feared social situations), specific phobia (e.g., on exposure to a specific phobic situation), obsessive-compulsive disorder (e.g., on exposure to dirt in someone with an obsession about contamination), posttraumatic stress disorder (e.g., in response to stimuli associated with a severe stressor), or separation anxiety disorder (e.g., in response to being away from home or close relatives).

Table 2–2.   DSM-IV-TR criteria for panic attack

Note: A panic attack is not a codable disorder. Code the specific diagnosis in which
   the panic attack occurs (e.g., 300.21 panic disorder with agoraphobia).

A discrete period of intense fear or discomfort, in which four (or more) of the following
   symptoms developed abruptly and reached a peak within 10 minutes:
   (1) palpitations, pounding heart, or accelerated heart rate
   (2) sweating
   (3) trembling or shaking
   (4) sensations of shortness of breath or smothering
   (5) feeling of choking
   (6) chest pain or discomfort
   (7) nausea or abdominal distress
   (8) feeling dizzy, unsteady, lightheaded, or faint
   (9) derealization (feelings of unreality) or depersonalization (being detached from
        oneself)
   (10) fear of losing control or going crazy
   (11) fear of dying
   (12) paresthesias (numbness or tingling sensations)
   (13) chills or hot flushes

Panic attacks are periods of intense fear, apprehension, or discomfort that
develop suddenly and reach a peak of intensity within 10 minutes of the initiation of symptoms. The DSM-IV-TR criteria require that four of 13 symptoms, including tachycardia, shortness of breath, and fear of dying or losing
control, be present for the diagnosis of a panic attack (Table 2–2). The sudden, often unexpected onset of panic attacks and their episodic nature distinguish them from the more diffuse symptoms characterizing anticipatory or
generalized anxiety. Indeed, panic attacks are not unique to panic disorder
and may occur in any of the anxiety disorders, on exposure to feared events.
Moreover, panic episodes may be reported by individuals not meeting criteria
for a specific anxiety disorder—occurring, for instance, during stressful situations.

Panic disorder was defined in DSM-III-R (American Psychiatric Association 1987) by the number of attacks (i.e., four) occurring over a 4-week
period. DSM-IV-TR eliminated the requirement for a specific number of attacks and emphasized the importance of the individual's phobic responses to
the panic episodes and their perceived consequences. In contrast, other disor-

ders may be characterized by panic responses that are situationally bound to phobic events, such as exposure to a social situation in social phobia or to a trauma cue in PTSD. Panic attacks that occur with fewer than four of the 13 panic symptoms specified by DSM-IV-TR are referred to as *limited-symptom attacks*. Most patients with panic disorder have a combination of full- and limited-symptom attacks.

In clinical settings, agoraphobia may be present in more three-quarters of patients with panic disorder (Breier et al. 1986). The term *agoraphobia* refers to a patient's fear, discomfort, or avoidance of situations in which escape may be difficult or help may not be readily available in the event of a panic attack (Table 2–3). Agoraphobic situations may include traveling on public transportation, going over bridges, being in open spaces or crowded places, standing in lines or in any situation in which the patient previously experienced a panic attack or from which easy escape is perceived as difficult. The severity of the agoraphobic avoidance may vary widely; some individuals, despite their fear and discomfort, push themselves through agoraphobic situations, whereas others may only endure them in the presence of a trusted companion or become literally homebound. For some individuals, the avoidance behavior may be cued by interoceptive or internal stimuli (e.g., rapid heart rate occurring during physical exercise or sexual arousal). Through fear conditioning, these stimuli may trigger a cognitive cascade of alarm and ultimately result in avoidance of the physical activity or situation linked to the distress.

Associated Features

The adverse impact of panic disorder on quality of life is comparable to that of major depression, and a number of studies have highlighted the adverse effect of panic disorder on multiple domains of function. One study reported that panic disorder is associated with a significant decrease in physical and mental functioning that is compounded in the presence of comorbid mood or anxiety disorders and is comparable to—and sometimes worse than—that in patients with chronic medical conditions and depression (Candilis et al. 1996). Panic disorder is associated with high rates of vocational dysfunction and financial dependence. Moreover, panic disorder is common in the general medical setting and is associated with increased use of health care services in affected individuals, with up to 13% of primary care patients having either panic disorder alone or the disorder combined with depression (Katon et al. 1986).

Table 2–3. DSM-IV-TR diagnostic criteria for agoraphobia

Note: Agoraphobia is not a codable disorder. Code the specific disorder in which the agoraphobia occurs (e.g., 300.21 panic disorder with agoraphobia or 300.22 agoraphobia without history of panic disorder).

A. Anxiety about being in places or situations from which escape might be difficult (or embarrassing) or in which help may not be available in the event of having an unexpected or situationally predisposed panic attack or panic-like symptoms. Agoraphobic fears typically involve characteristic clusters of situations that include being outside the home alone; being in a crowd or standing in a line; being on a bridge; and traveling in a bus, train, or automobile.

Note: Consider the diagnosis of specific phobia if the avoidance is limited to one or only a few specific situations, or social phobia if the avoidance is limited to social situations.

B. The situations are avoided (e.g., travel is restricted) or else are endured with marked distress or with anxiety about having a panic attack or panic-like symptoms, or require the presence of a companion.

C. The anxiety or phobic avoidance is not better accounted for by another mental disorder, such as social phobia (e.g., avoidance limited to social situations because of fear of embarrassment), specific phobia (e.g., avoidance limited to a single situation like elevators), obsessive-compulsive disorder (e.g., avoidance of dirt in someone with an obsession about contamination), posttraumatic stress disorder (e.g., avoidance of stimuli associated with a severe stressor), or separation anxiety disorder (e.g., avoidance of leaving home or relatives).

Like other psychiatric conditions, panic disorder is often unrecognized and untreated in primary care settings, as illustrated by a World Health Organization primary care study that found that the diagnosis of panic was missed in half of all affected patients (Sartorius et al. 1993). Underrecognition may, in part, be attributable to the typical presentation of patients with panic disorder and the predominantly somatic (i.e., chest pain, dizziness, shortness of breath, irritable bowel) rather than psychological symptoms. Analysis of data from the Epidemiologic Catchment Area (ECA) study revealed that patients with panic disorder were five to eight times more likely than nonaffected individuals to be frequent users of medical services (Simon and VonKorff 1991). Prompt and early recognition and treatment of panic disorder in general medical settings is critical, as treatment results in symptomatic relief, improvement in role functioning, decreased use of medical resources, and reduction in overall costs. In addition, there is evidence suggesting that panic disorder may be associated with increased risk for death from cardiovascular causes (Kawachi et al. 1994). Studies suggest that pharmacotherapy for panic disorder normalizes the decreased heart rate variability hypothesized to contribute to excessive cardiac mortality associated with panic (Tucker et al. 1997).

Epidemiology

Panic disorder was not defined as a distinct entity until the publication of DSM-III (American Psychiatric Association 1980); therefore, there are few, if any, specific data on its epidemiology prior to that point. The lifetime prevalence of panic attacks and panic disorder has been estimated through a series of epidemiological studies, including the National Institute of Mental Health ECA Program and the National Comorbidity Survey (NCS) (Kessler et al. 1994).

The lifetime prevalence of panic attacks in the ECA study, as defined using DSM-III criteria (including four or more psychophysiological symptoms), was 9.7%. The NCS estimate, using similar criteria, was 15.6%; however, when the definition for panic attack was more narrowly defined using DSM-III-R criteria (American Psychiatric Association 1987), its prevalence dropped to 7.3%. The lifetime prevalence of panic disorder ranged from 1.7% in the ECA study to 3.5% in the NCS; the 1-month prevalence was 0.5% in the ECA study and 1.5% in the NCS. Differences in the reported prevalence of panic disorder between the studies may be accounted for by the slightly different target populations and the methodologies (the ECA study interviewed patients age 18 years and older; the NCS was a nationwide survey of men and women between the ages of 15 and 54 years) and also by the diagnostic criteria used in each study (the ECA used DSM-III criteria as determined by the Diagnostic Interview Schedule; the NCS used DSM-III-R criteria as determined by the Composite International Diagnostic Interview).

Panic disorder is more commonly diagnosed in women than in men, with a 3:1 ratio in patients with agoraphobia and 2:1 ratio in patients without agoraphobia. Although on average the onset of panic disorder is in the third decade, approximately one-half of adult patients report significant anxiety during childhood, in the form of overanxious disorder, social phobia, or separation anxiety disorder (Pollack et al. 1996a). Although the onset of panic may be spontaneous, many individuals identify a life stressor occurring prior to the onset of panic symptoms (Manfro et al. 1996).

Although agoraphobia without panic disorder may occur even more commonly than panic disorder with agoraphobia in the community, it is much less common among clinical populations. Clinical reevaluation of subjects with diagnosed agoraphobia without panic disorder in community surveys indicates that many have specific phobia rather than agoraphobia.

Assessment

Differential Diagnosis

Patients with panic disorder tend to report multiple physical symptoms across different organ systems, complicating their diagnosis, particularly in general medical settings. The distinction between *panic disorder, somatization disorders*, and *hypochondriasis* may thus be complex. Patients with somatoform disorders may have a history of physical or sexual abuse, a history of alcohol or substance abuse, and a pattern of maladaptive interpersonal relationships that may assist in differentiating them from patients with panic disorder. Panic disorder may be complicated by the presence of comorbid conditions, including other anxiety disorders (e.g., social phobia, generalized anxiety disorder, PTSD, obsessive-compulsive disorder [OCD]), depression, and alcohol abuse.

Social phobia may occur in up to one-third of patients with panic disorder. Differentiating panic and social phobia may sometimes be difficult, particularly when panic attacks occur in social situations. The focus of the patient's core fears may help make the diagnosis; in panic disorder, the central fear is of having a panic attack and may manifest in situations outside of social ones. Patients with social phobia, who have panic episodes on exposure to social scrutiny, focus primarily on the possibility of humiliation or embarrassment in social situations. For many patients, both types of fears may be present and the diagnosis of both conditions is then warranted.

Generalized anxiety disorder (GAD) is also frequently comorbid with panic disorder. Occasionally, the excessive worry and anxiety associated with GAD may become acutely intense and associated with physical symptoms that resemble a panic attack. Patients with GAD, however, worry excessively about life events or stressors, whereas those with panic disorder focus on anticipation of recurrent panic attacks.

Patients with *specific phobias*, *PTSD*, and *OCD* may also experience panic attacks, but these are typically cued by exposure to or anticipation of specific phobic situations (e.g., contamination in patients with OCD, heights or other phobic situations in patients with specific phobias, and trauma-related events in PTSD). For individuals with these conditions, panic attacks are rarely unexpected or spontaneous unless panic disorder is also present.

Among the most common comorbid conditions associated with panic disorder is *depression*, with up to two-thirds of panic disorder patients experiencing major depression at some point during their life. Depression may either predate or emerge after the onset of panic disorder and may reflect either a reactive demoralization related to the negative effects of panic or the emergence of an independent condition. As is true with other comorbid conditions, the presence of comorbid depression may complicate treatment and increase the overall severity of the patient's distress. The presence of panic attacks in patients with major depression is associated with an increased risk of suicide (Fawcett et al. 1990). Although data from the ECA study suggested an increased risk of suicide associated with panic disorder alone (Weissman et al. 1989), evaluation of this issue in clinical populations suggests that the risk is elevated predominantly in panic disorder patients with comorbid depression and/or personality dysfunction (Cox et al. 1994).

Alcohol abuse and dependence may also be present in up to one-quarter of individuals with panic disorder. Although some individuals report that their abuse of alcohol developed in the context of an attempt to self-medicate their anxiety, the temporal relationship between alcohol abuse and panic disorder tends to follow the typical ages of onset for the disorders, with the mean onset of alcohol abuse occurring in the late teens to early 20s and of panic disorder in the late 20s (Otto et al. 1992a). Clinically, the presence of alcohol abuse should be considered in all individuals presenting with panic and other anxiety disorders and may represent a relative contraindication to the use of benzodiazepines (BZs); patients abusing alcohol or drugs typically require focused substance abuse treatment, in addition to anxiolytic therapy, to achieve comprehensive recovery.

The differential diagnosis of panic disorder in the medical setting also includes a number of medical conditions and the drugs used to treat them. Thyroid disease, cardiac arrhythmias, pheochromocytoma, autonomic disorders, asthma, congestive heart failure, chronic obstructive pulmonary disease, mitral valve prolapse, orthostatic hypotension, parathyroid dysfunction, seizure disorder, pulmonary embolism, angina, and transient ischemic attacks may resemble panic disorder. In addition, use of caffeine, cannabis, amphetamines, and cocaine, or withdrawal from alcohol or sedatives, may result in panic-like symptoms.

Assessment Measures

The goal of diagnostic assessment is to confirm the presence of panic disorder and to investigate comorbid conditions that may influence its presentation and course. The severity and frequency of panic attacks may vary widely, with patients experiencing episodes anywhere between once a month and daily. Historically, assessment of severity and treatment response in panic disorder was based almost exclusively on the frequency and intensity of panic attacks. However, frequency may be a misleading indicator of the true severity of the condition, as some patients may reduce the frequency by avoiding situations that trigger them. Thus, a consensus conference on the assessment of panic disorder recommended broadening the domain of symptoms evaluated to include not just panic disorder frequency and severity but also phobic anxiety, avoidance, and interference with function (Shear and Maser 1994). The Panic Disorder Severity Scale is a seven-item scale developed to assess these aspects of the panic disorder syndrome and their change with treatment (Shear et al. 1997). Instruments such as the Sheehan Disability Scale (Sheehan 1983), the Medical Outcome Study Short Form-36 (Ware and Sherbourne 1992), and the Quality of Life Enjoyment and Satisfaction Questionnaire (Endicott et al. 1993) are also used to measure quality of life and functional impairment and their treatment response in patients with panic disorder.

Pathogenesis

Understanding of the neurobiology of panic disorder has undergone unprecedented growth since the groundbreaking studies of Klein in the early 1960s (Klein and Fink 1962). Recent developments in neuroimaging and molecular genetics have bolstered further advances, though many crucial questions remain unanswered. Although the following section should not be regarded as comprehensive, we summarize some pertinent aspects of the neurobiology of panic disorder (Coplan and Lydiard 1998; Gorman et al. 2000).

Neurochemistry

A substantial body of evidence suggests that panic disorder is associated with dysfunction of brain monoaminergic systems (i.e., the noradenergic [norepinephrine; NE] and serotonin [5-hydroxytryptamine; 5-HT] systems), the GABA (γ-aminobutyric acid) system, and respiratory and cardiovascular functions.

Norepinephrine

The noradrenergic system has been implicated in the pathophysiology of fear and anxiety behavior, including panic disorder (Redmond et al. 1976). The locus coeruleus, the major NE-containing brain structure, receives afferent information from the sensory system and sends efferents to several brain areas involved in the fear network, including the amygdala, cortex, hippocampus, and hypothalamus. Preclinical studies suggest that the NE system is stress-responsive and mediates fear conditioning (Abercrombie and Jacobs 1987). Furthermore, the central and peripheral NE systems seem to function independently, perhaps indicating how either internal or external cues can trigger panic attacks. Patients with panic disorder demonstrated increased noradrenergic activity, with responses to pharmacological challenges of noradrenergic agents, suggesting presynaptic α_2-adrenoreceptor dysregulation and increased peripheral β-adrenoreceptor sensitivity. The responsiveness of panic symptoms to pharmacological agents such as tricyclic antidepressants (TCAs) and monoamine oxidase inhibitors (MAOIs) that modulate NE function also underscores the likely role of NE in the pathogenesis of panic disorder.

Serotonin

Studies support the involvement of 5-HT in the pathophysiology of panic disorder, although its precise role has yet to be determined (Grove et al. 1997). Regardless, the well-established clinical efficacy of serotonergic agents such as selective serotonin reuptake inhibitors (SSRIs) in the treatment of panic disorder and evidence of serotonergic regulation of the NE system offer additional insight into possible mechanisms through which the 5-HT system is relevant.

Benzodiazepines and GABA

BZs such as alprazolam and clonazepam block panic attacks and are established pharmacological treatments for panic disorder. Flumazenil, a BZ antagonist, induces panic attacks in patients with panic disorder but not in healthy subjects (Nutt et al. 1990). These findings suggest a possible BZ receptor abnormality or deficiency of a structurally similar endogenous substance, although this remains speculative. Additional lines of evidence suggesting a potential role of the GABA system in the pathogenesis of panic disorder include the observation that agents such as valproic acid and gabapentin that affect the GABAergic system appear to effectively treat panic symptoms. In addition, low plasma GABA levels may be associated with a less robust response to adequate antipanic treatment (Rimon et al. 1995). Furthermore, inhibition of GABA synthesis produces increased anxiety sensitivity in animal models (Shekhar et al. 1996).

Lactate and Carbon Dioxide Metabolism

Extensive literature supports the panicogenic effects of both lactate and carbon dioxide (CO_2) in patients with panic disorder (Klein 1993). Lactate- and CO_2-induced panic attacks can be blocked by a variety of pharmacological and cognitive-behavioral interventions effective for the treatment of panic disorder. Voluntary hyperventilation has been reported to trigger panic attacks and is known to cause hypocapnia and also increased brain lactate levels. In addition, there is evidence suggesting that both hypercapnia and hypocapnia may induce panic attacks. Thus, it has been hypothesized that fluctuations in brain CO_2 and pH levels may elicit panic episodes by activating a suffocation false-alarm response in susceptible individuals (Klein 1993). Some studies have demonstrated that patients with panic disorder seem to have abnormal sensitivity to these fluctuations. However, the biochemical mechanisms underlying the panicogenic effects of lactate and CO_2 remain unclear.

Cardiovascular Function

Cardiovascular and autonomic symptoms of arousal are hallmarks of panic attacks. A number of studies in patients with panic disorder have documented decreased heart rate variability (HRV—i.e., beat-to-beat variation) secondary to predominant sympathetic activation and decreased vagal tone; this may in turn contribute to the increased susceptibility to malignant arrhythmias and thus morbidity and mortality in patients with panic disorder (Kawachi et al.

1995). Although lactate and isoproterenol can exaggerate reductions in HRV in these patients, effective panic treatment appears to normalize HRV in panic (Tucker et al. 1997).

Neuroanatomy

Amygdala

Converging lines of data link the amygdala to fear and anxiety behaviors. Stimulation of the amygdala elicits fearlike behaviors and physiological arousal in animals. Conversely, ablation of the amygdala interferes with the acquisition of conditioned fear (Davis 1992). In addition, evidence suggests that the amygdala has a significant role in determining emotional responses to sensory stimuli (Le Doux 1992).

Locus Coeruleus

As noted above, numerous lines of evidence support the involvement of noradrenergic systems, and its principal nucleus in the human brain, the locus coeruleus, with development of fear and anxiety. Electrical and other stimulation of the locus coeruleus produces fear in animal models, whereas bilateral lesions result in attenuation of fear and anxiety behavior (Redmond et al. 1976). In addition, exposure to threatening situations increases activity in the locus coeruleus.

Other Structures

Several other central nervous system (CNS) structures have been implicated in the underlying neurophysiology of fear and anxiety, including the thalamus and hypothalamus, the hippocampus, the anterior cingulate gyrus, the periaqueductal gray area, and the frontal cortex. Emerging evidence suggests that a neuronal network involving the hippocampus, the cortex, and the amygdala may function in contextual conditioning secondary to fear stimuli (Gorman et al. 2000).

Neuroimaging

Growing evidence from neuroimaging studies suggests that CNS structural and functional abnormalities are implicated in the pathogenesis of panic disorder (Gorman et al. 2000). However, interpretation of some of these findings is obscured because it remains unclear whether detected abnormalities (e.g., in anterior cingulate function) reflect the pathogenesis of panic or represent normal anxiety states. Nonetheless, positron emission tomography and single-photon emission computed tomography studies demonstrate increased cerebral blood flow during fear conditioning in the thalamus, hypothalamus, periaqueductal gray region, cingulate, and somatosensory and associative cortex, supporting their involvement in the fear network. Functional magnetic resonance imaging studies have demonstrated activation of the amygdala and periamygdaloid cortical areas during conditioned fear and extinction and also in response to exposure to affectively negative or fearful visual stimuli (LaBar et al. 1998). In addition, one study demonstrated a strong increase in amygdala activity in response to CO_2 inhalation (Corfield et al. 1995).

Pharmacotherapy

The goals of the treatment of panic disorder are to significantly reduce or eliminate panic attacks, avoidance, and anticipatory anxiety and to treat any comorbid conditions. The effectiveness of both pharmacotherapy and cognitive-behavioral therapy for panic disorder has been established in well-controlled clinical studies. Selection of treatment modality should include review of the risks and benefits of each therapeutic intervention and consideration of patients' preferences. In addition, the presence of relevant comorbidities may help guide the selection of an appropriate intervention—for instance, patients with panic disorder and significant comorbid depression should generally receive therapy with an antidepressant, whereas BZ administration should be avoided if possible in those with comorbid substance abuse.

Antidepressants

Selective Serotonin Reuptake Inhibitors

SSRIs have become a first-line pharmacotherapy for mood and anxiety disorders, including panic disorder. There is now convincing evidence for the efficacy of each of the available SSRIs, including fluvoxamine (150–300 mg/day), paroxetine (40–60 mg/day), controlled-release paroxetine (25–75 mg/day), fluoxetine (10–20 mg/day), sertraline (50–200 mg /day), citalopram (20–40 mg/day), and escitalopram (10–40 mg/day), in the acute and long-term treatment of panic disorder (Sheehan and Harnett-Sheehan 1996). Clomipramine may be the most effective TCA for the treatment of panic disorder, perhaps because of its more potent serotonergic properties (Modigh et al. 1992). However, the SSRIs appear to be at least as efficacious as clomipramine in comparative trials and are generally better tolerated.

Individuals with panic disorder are particularly sensitive to the activating effects associated with initiation of SSRIs and other antidepressants, such as insomnia, restlessness, jitteriness, and agitation. Should these adverse effects occur without prior patient preparation, early treatment discontinuation may result. As with the TCAs, SSRI treatment should be initiated at low doses (e.g., 10 mg/day paroxetine or 12.5 mg/day of controlled-release preparation; 25 mg/day sertraline; 25 mg/day fluvoxamine; 10 mg/day fluoxetine; 10 mg/day citalopram; or 5–10 mg/day escitalopram) with gradual upward titration.

Compared with the older classes of antidepressants, including TCAs and MAOIs, therapy with SSRIs is associated with less weight gain, fewer or absent anticholinergic effects, a relatively benign cardiovascular profile (e.g., no orthostatic dizziness or cardiac conduction effects), and safety in overdose. However, SSRI-associated side effects, including gastrointestinal distress and sexual dysfunction, may be problematic for some patients.

Tricyclic Antidepressants

The majority of the information regarding the use of TCAs for panic disorder is derived from studies of imipramine and clomipramine. In almost all studies, imipramine and clomipramine are superior to placebo. One study reported that clomipramine was more effective than imipramine (Modigh et al. 1992). Clomipramine is often prescribed at doses of 150–200 mg/day but has been shown to be effective for at least some patients at lower doses (25–50 mg daily) (Gloger et al. 1989). Other studies indicate that the TCAs desipramine and nortriptyline are also effective for panic disorder (Lydiard and Ballenger 1987). However, because TCAs are associated with a significant side effect burden over the longer term, have substantial toxicity in overdose, and lack efficacy for some comorbid disorders commonly occurring with panic disorder, such as social phobia, they have been supplanted by SSRIs as first-line pharmacotherapy.

Monoamine Oxidase Inhibitors

The irreversible MAOIs phenelzine and tranylcypromine appear at least as effective as TCAs for the treatment of panic disorder. In fact, some clinicians believe them to be the most comprehensively effective agents for the treatment of depression and anxiety disorders, although there are no definitive data addressing this issue. In addition, there are no studies to date comparing SSRIs and MAOIs for panic disorder. The aversive side effect profile of

MAOIs, however, including weight gain, orthostatic hypotension, and sexual dysfunction, is a significant disadvantage. In addition, the need for dietary tyramine restriction and the risk of hypertensive crisis further limit the broad usefulness of these agents for panic disorder. It was once hoped that selective reversible inhibitors of monoamine oxidase type A, such as brofaromine (van Vliet et al. 1996) and moclobemide (Kruger and Dahl 1999), which have a more favorable side effects profile than standard MAOIs and entail no need for tyramine restriction, represented an advance for the treatment of panic disorder. However, results of controlled trials with these agents are equivocal overall, and neither is available in the United States, although moclobemide is available in some countries.

Other Antidepressants

Some of the other newer antidepressants, including venlafaxine (Pollack et al. 1996b), nefazodone (Papp et al. 2000), and mirtazapine (Boshuisen et al. 2001), have demonstrated potential efficacy in smaller studies of panic disorder and, with their distinct mechanisms of action and side effect profiles, diversify the available therapeutic options. Bupropion has been generally considered ineffective for the treatment of panic disorder on the basis of negative findings of one study (Sheehan et al. 1983). However, clinical experience and a more recent study (Emmanuel et al. 2000) suggest that it may, in fact, have antipanic efficacy and that additional research with this agent is warranted.

Benzodiazepines

Although the "pharmacological dissection" of anxiety posited that BZs were ineffective for the treatment of panic, a number of large placebo-controlled studies done primarily during the 1980s demonstrated the high-potency BZ alprazolam to be superior to placebo in treating patients with panic disorder or agoraphobia with panic attacks (Ballenger et al. 1988). Alprazolam was the first drug approved by the U.S. Food and Drug Administration for treatment of panic disorder. Because of alprazolam's relative short duration of action, treatment with the drug requires dosing three to four times daily for many patients.

Observations of interdose rebound anxiety, presumably due to fluctuations in alprazolam plasma levels during treatment (Herman et al. 1987), prompted evaluation of the use of BZs with longer durations of action such as clonazepam. In a placebo-controlled trial, clonazepam was shown to be as effective for panic disorder as alprazolam (Tesar et al. 1991). Furthermore, its longer elimination half-life (20–50 hours) permitted once or twice daily dosing for most patients. Although agents with longer elimination half-lives were believed to be more easily tapered off than shorter-acting agents, this appears to be true primarily only with abrupt discontinuation.

Controlled studies suggest that the rate of BZ taper may be the critical determinant of the success of discontinuation efforts, with a gradual taper eliminating differences in emergent withdrawal difficulties between short- and long-acting agents (Rickels et al. 1990). Administration of CBT directed at control of symptoms during BZ discontinuation has been helpful for some patients as well (Otto et al. 1993). Despite the earlier belief that potency is a critical determinant of antipanic efficacy, the evidence suggests that all BZs, including lorazepam and diazepam, can be effective if administered at equipotent doses (Noyes et al. 1996).

BZs have the advantage of excellent tolerability and more rapid onset of action compared to antidepressants. However, their use is associated with the development of dependence with regular use, and abuse liability in predisposed individuals. In addition, BZs are not generally effective for depression, which often presents comorbidly with panic disorder.

Anticonvulsants

Valproic acid is a mood-stabilizing anticonvulsant that has been reported in small studies to be effective for the treatment of panic disorder (Woodman and Noyes 1994). As an anticonvulsant mood stabilizer, it may be particularly useful for patients with panic disorder and concurrent seizures or bipolar disorder. Conversely, carbamazepine appears to be ineffective for panic disorder (Uhde et al. 1988). Gabapentin is another anticonvulsant that appears to have anxiolytic effects and has been demonstrated effective in a placebo-controlled double-blind study for the treatment of panic disorder (600–3,600 mg/day) (Pande et al. 2000).

Other Agents

Buspirone, a partial serotonin 5-HT$_{1A}$ receptor agonist, does not appear to be effective as a primary treatment for panic disorder (Sheehan et al. 1993), although reports suggest that it may sometimes be used as an adjunct to antidepressants and BZs (Gastfriend and Rosenbaum 1989). Sometimes used as anxiolytics, particularly in primary care settings, β-blockers (e.g., propranolol) do not actually appear to be useful as first-line agents for panic disorder, although they, too, may be useful as adjunctive agents. They reduce symptoms of autonomic arousal, such as tachycardia and tremor, but do not treat the cognitive or emotional experience of anxiety. Table 2–4 summarizes the usual dose range of pharmacological agents used for the treatment of panic disorder.

Maintenance Pharmacotherapy

The efficacy of short-term pharmacological treatment for panic disorder has been confirmed with a number of pharmacological agents, such BZs, TCAs, SSRIs, and MAOIs. However, there have been limited controlled research studies examining the long-term treatment, course, and outcome of panic disorder. Naturalistic data suggest that panic disorder has a chronic, relapsing course for many patients (Pollack and Marzol 2000). Typical response rates for TCA and BZ long-term treatment range from 50% to 70%, with remission rates of 20% to 50% and relapse rates of 25% to 85% after treatment discontinuation (Pollack and Otto 1997). Mavissakalian and Perel (1992) examined whether a longer duration of maintenance treatment with TCAs would promote a lower relapse rate. They found that patients who received imipramine for 18 months after acute response had a lower rate of relapse after medication discontinuation than those receiving imipramine for only 6 months. Replication of this finding with SSRIs remains to be done, but these results suggest that treatment should be maintained for at least 1–2 years after response to decrease the risk of relapse after treatment discontinuation.

Although most patients' symptoms decrease with treatment, many patients remain at least somewhat symptomatic. In long-term observations (1.5–6 years), approximately 30%–80% of patients continue to experience panic attacks, anticipatory anxiety, and/or avoidance behavior after initiating treatment. In a naturalistic study of patients with panic disorder treated with a variety of pharmacotherapies, nearly one-half (46.2%) of patients who initially achieved remission had a relapse within a 24-month follow-up period, with a mean time to relapse of 6 months (Simon et al. 2002), despite continued treatment. Recent studies examined longer-term use of SSRIs for panic, although the period of observation may still be too relatively brief to fully inform clinical practice. In one study, patients were randomly assigned, after acute paroxetine treatment, to placebo or continued paroxetine for an addi-

Table 2–4. Commonly prescribed antipanic agents

Drug	Daily dosage range (mg)	Initial dose (mg)	Dosing schedule
Selective serotonin reuptake inhibitors			
Paroxetine	10–60	10	qd
Controlled-release paroxetine	25–75	12.5	qd
Sertraline	25–200	25	qd
Fluoxetine	10–80	10	qd
Citalopram	20–60	10	qd
Escitalopram	10–40	5–10	qd
Fluvoxamine	100–300	50	qd
Tricyclic antidepressants			
Imipramine	100–300	10–25	qd
Clomipramine	100–250	12.5–25	qd
Monoamine oxidase inhibitors			
Phenelzine	45–90	15	bid
Tranylcypromine	30–60	10	bid
Other antidepressants			
Mirtazapine	15–45	7.5	qd
Nefazodone	100–600	50	bid
Venlafaxine	75–375	37.5	qd
Other agents			
Buspirone	15–60	5	bid–tid
Valproic acid	500–2,000	250	bid
Gabapentin	900–3,600	300	tid
Benzodiazepines			
Alprazolam	2–6	0.25–0.5	tid–qid
Clonazepam	1–5	0.5	bid
Lorazepam	3–9	0.5–1	tid–qid
Diazepam	5–60	2.5	bid

tional 12 weeks. Thirty percent of patients who switched to a placebo had a relapse, whereas only 5% of those who continued to take paroxetine had a relapse (Lydiard et al. 1998). Similarly, rates of relapse in a study following patients after acute treatment with fluoxetine reported a relapse rate of 3% for those who continued taking the SSRI for an additional 22 weeks (Michelson et al. 1999). In a 52-week open-label sertraline trial followed by a 28-week double-blind placebo-controlled discontinuation period, symptom exacerbation occurred in 33% of placebo-treated patients, compared with 13% of patients who continued to take sertraline (Rapaport et al. 2001). Further research is warranted to establish the optimal length of treatment continuation and to identify patients who may be able to successfully discontinue treatment and those who would benefit from ongoing maintenance therapy.

Treatment-Refractory Panic Disorder

To facilitate the development of interventions for patients who remain symptomatic after initial treatment, it is important to determine the reason for treatment failure. Factors that may contribute to the persistence of symptoms include concurrent depression, other comorbid anxiety conditions, concomitant personality disorders, severe agoraphobia at baseline, and frequent and severe panic attacks at baseline (Cowley et al. 1997). Cowley and colleagues reported that intolerance to side effects was the most common reason for treatment failure, occurring in 27% of the population assessed, which consisted largely of patients taking TCAs. Other issues that should be considered include substance abuse, noncompliance, inadequate dose or treatment duration, medical illness, misdiagnosis, and inappropriate medication selection (Simon and Pollack 1999).

Limited information on treatment for patients with panic disorder who remain symptomatic despite initial treatment is available in the literature (Scott et al. 1999). There are several reviews offering recommendations, open case series and case reports describing combination strategies for patients with treatment-refractory panic disorder. These preliminary reports suggest that adjunctive use of agents such as valproate (Ontiveros and Fontaine 1992), gabapentin (Pollack et al. 1998), β-blockers, and buspirone (Gastfriend and Rosenbaum 1989) may provide additional relief of panic-related anxiety symptoms. Addition of a TCA to an SSRI has also been suggested to be a useful strategy (Tiffon et al. 1994). One small placebo-controlled trial in patients with treatment-refractory panic disorder demonstrated the efficacy of pindolol as an augmentation strategy (Hirschmann et al. 2000).

Psychotherapy

Recent decades have brought significant advances in the psychosocial treatments of panic disorder and agoraphobia, including cognitive-behavioral, psychodynamic, and interpersonal therapies. In particular, cognitive-behavioral therapy (CBT) has been refined by Barlow and others (Barlow and Craske 1994) to focus on interoceptive exposure to somatic arousal and other sensations that may cue panic—in contrast to more traditional CBT, which focuses primarily on in vivo exposure to specific situations associated with panic attacks and agoraphobia.

Cognitive-Behavioral Therapy

Cognitive-Behavioral Model of Panic Disorder

According to the cognitive-behavioral model of panic disorder, panic attacks are considered a manifestation of the fight-or-flight alarm system that may sometimes initially emerge during or after a period of stress. As such alarm reactions occur unexpectedly and in the absence of external danger, they may become the objects of fear themselves. Catastrophic misinterpretations of the meaning of the somatic sensations that accompany the panic attacks evoke fears of death, insanity, disease, social embarrassment, and disability. With each attack, the anxiety and resultant fear anticipating the next episode leads to heightened anxiety levels, physiological arousal, and focus on the feared bodily sensations that consequently cue repeated attacks, thus creating a self-maintained cycle. The "fear-of-fear cycle" is summarized in Figure 2–1 (Otto et al. 1992b), underscoring the role of conditioned fear, bodily symptoms, and catastrophic cognitions in the pathogenesis and perpetuation of panic disorder.

Treatment Components and Effectiveness of Cognitive-Behavioral Therapy

Several versions of CBT for panic disorder have been developed. The most well studied and commonly used is known as *panic control treatment* (PCT) (Barlow and Craske 1994). PCT consists of the following components: education about the nature of anxiety and panic, identification and correction of maladaptive thoughts about anxiety and its consequences (cognitive restructuring), training in arousal-reduction techniques such as diaphragmatic slow breathing (breathing retraining), and graded exposure to bodily sensations

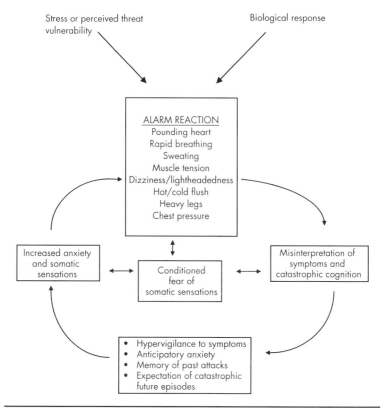

Figure 2–1.   Fear-of-fear cycle.
Source. Adapted from Otto MW, Pollack MH, Meltzer-Brody S, et al.: "Cognitive-Behavioral Therapy for Benzodiazepine Discontinuation in Panic Disorder Patients." *Psychopharmacology Bulletin* 28(2):123–130, 1992. Reprinted with permission.

that resemble those experienced during anxiety and panic (interoceptive or structured exposure). Treatment is usually delivered in 12 to 15 sessions over a period of 3 to 4 months (Barlow and Craske 1994).

The efficacy of PCT has been demonstrated in numerous studies (Barlow et al. 1989). Studies comparing PCT to other standard panic treatments report comparable or higher response rates. For instance, in one study, PCT was compared with alprazolam, placebo, and a wait-list control. In the PCT group, 87% of CBT-treated patients were panic-free by the end of treatment, compared with 50% in the alprazolam group, 36% in the placebo group, and 33% on the wait list (Klosko et al. 1995). In another study of 8 weeks' duration, 85% of PCT patients were panic-free, versus 30% in a wait-list control condition (Telch et al. 1993).

Combined Treatments

Although combining pharmacotherapy and psychosocial interventions is common in clinical practice, it is not clear whether combined treatment is more effective than either pharmacotherapy or CBT alone for most patients.

A recent survey of experts on the pharmacological treatment of anxiety found that most favored combined treatment for panic disorder (Uhlenhuth 1998); however, clinical studies of combined treatments have not consistently found significant advantages over monotherapy. One of the earliest rationales for combining pharmacotherapy and psychosocial treatments for panic disorder was Klein's (1980) suggestion that drugs might work preferentially to suppress panic attacks whereas exposure therapy more specifically addresses agoraphobic avoidance. In accordance with that suggestion, a number of studies have been conducted comparing the effect of combined drug (antidepressants or BZs) and exposure treatments against one or both treatments alone (Barlow et al. 2000). Overall, these studies show modest, short-term advantages for the combination of antidepressants and CBT over either treatment alone, whereas some of the available data on combining BZs and exposure therapy indicate worse long-term outcomes for the combined treatment than for CBT alone (Otto et al. 1996). The possible detrimental effect of BZs on the outcome of CBT appears to be minimized if the drugs are discontinued prior to the conclusion of CBT.

Recently, a multicenter trial comparing imipramine, CBT, and their combination demonstrated that in the acute (3 months) and maintenance (6 months of follow-up) treatment of panic, response rates were equivalent for the CBT and imipramine groups, with both superior to rates for placebo (Barlow et al. 2000). The results for CBT plus imipramine were similar to those for CBT plus placebo in the acute period; however, the former regimen gained superiority during the 6-month maintenance phase. In the 6 months after imipramine discontinuation, responders to CBT alone or CBT plus placebo had a better outcome than those whose disorder responded to imipramine with or without CBT. This study suggested that combined treatment may have some modest additional benefit above monotherapy during 6 months of treatment, whereas CBT may have more durable maintenance of gains after treatment discontinuation.

On the basis of the available evidence, it appears that routine initial administration of pharmacotherapy with CBT is not warranted in most instances. Whether there are some patients for whom such an approach would be indicated is not known at present. For now, the greatest support for combining treatments is for the addition of in vivo exposure therapy to pharmacotherapy for patients with agoraphobia (Mavissakalian 1993) and for the administration of CBT to patients attempting medication discontinuation (Otto et al. 1993).

Psychodynamic Psychotherapies

Although there is limited empirical research demonstrating the efficacy of psychodynamic therapies for panic disorder, such interventions are often used in practice. Preliminary studies and case reports indicate that psychodynamic psychotherapies can be efficacious for the treatment of panic disorder. A recent open trial on the treatment of panic disorder using a manualized psychodynamic approach known as *panic-focused psychodynamic psychotherapy* showed improvement in symptoms and quality of life, suggesting it as a promising option (Milrod et al. 2001). One study investigating the effect of adding psychodynamic psychotherapy to clomipramine showed that relapse rates after discontinuation were lower than those with clomipramine alone (Wilborg and Dahl 1996). However, a controlled study using emotion-focused psychodynamic psychotherapy found it to be comparable to placebo and less effective than either CBT or imipramine for panic disorder (Shear et al. 2001). Further investigation of the use of psychodynamic psychotherapy as monotherapy and as an augmentation strategy for patients receiving CBT or pharmacotherapy may clarify the role of more psychodynamically oriented psychotherapeutic approaches for the treatment of panic disorder.

Conclusion

The recognition, assessment, and treatment of panic disorder have greatly advanced over the past several years. Increased understanding of the underlying pathophysiology of panic disorder will likely be obtained through neuroimaging, molecular, and genomics research. As the distress and impairment associated with panic have become more widely appreciated, the need for effective treatment has also become clearer. Thus, the current challenge in panic disorder research is to further refine diagnostic and assessment tools and to identify more effective, safe, and well-tolerated treatments that produce resolution of symptoms and promote establishment of optimal function and quality of life in affected individuals.

References

Abercrombie ED, Jacobs BL: Single-unit response of noradrenergic neurons in the locus coeruleus of freely moving cats, I: acutely presented stressful and nonstressful stimuli. J Neurosci 7:2837–2843, 1987

American Psychiatric Association: Diagnostic and Statistical Manual of Mental Disorders, 3rd Edition. Washington, DC, American Psychiatric Association, 1980

American Psychiatric Association: Diagnostic and Statistical Manual of Mental Disorders, 3rd Edition, Revised. Washington, DC, American Psychiatric Association, 1987

American Psychiatric Association: Diagnostic and Statistical Manual of Mental Disorders, 4th Edition, Text Revision. Washington, DC, American Psychiatric Association, 2000

Ballenger JC, Burrows GD, DuPont RL Jr, et al: Alprazolam in panic disorder and agoraphobia: results from a multicenter trial, I: efficacy in short-term treatment. Arch Gen Psychiatry 45: 413–422, 1988

Barlow DH, Craske MG: Mastery of Your Anxiety and Panic, 2nd Edition (MAP II). Albany, NY, Graywind Publications, 1994

Barlow DH, Craske MG, Cerny JA, et al: Behavioral treatment of panic disorder. Behav Ther 20:261–282, 1989

Barlow DH, Gorman JM, Shear MK, et al: Cognitive-behavioral therapy, imipramine, or their combination for panic disorder: a randomized controlled trial. JAMA 283:2529–2536, 2000

Boshuisen ML, Slaap BR, Vester-Blokland ED, et al: The effect of mirtazapine in panic disorder: an open label pilot study with a single-blind placebo run-in period. Int Clin Psychopharmacol 16:363–368, 2001

Breier A, Charney D, Heninger G: Agoraphobia with panic attacks: Development, diagnostic stability, and course of illness. Arch Gen Psychiatry 43:1029–1036, 1986

Candilis PJ, Manfro GG, Worthington JJ, et al: General and mental health function in panic disorder. Poster presented at the 16th annual conference of the Anxiety Disorders Association of America, Orlando, FL, March 1996

Coplan JD, Lydiard RB: Brain circuits in panic disorder. Biol Psychiatry 44:1264–1276, 1998

Corfield DR, Fink GR, Ramsay SC, et al: Activation of limbic structures during CO_2-stimulated breathing in awake man, in Modeling and Control of Ventilation. Edited by Semple SJG, Adams L, Whipp BJ. New York, Plenum, 1995, pp 331–334

Cowley DS, Ha EH, Roy-Byrne PP: Determinants of pharmacologic treatment failure in panic disorder. J Clin Psychiatry. 58:555–561, 1997

Cox BJ, Doremfeld DM, Swinson RP, et al: Suicidal ideation and suicide attempts in panic disorder and social phobia. Am J Psychiatry 151:882–887, 1994

Davis M: The role of the amygdala in fear and anxiety. Annu Rev Neurosci 15:353–375, 1992

Emmanuel NP, Pollack MH, Morton AW, et al: Bupropion-sustained release in the treatment of panic disorder. Poster presented at the 41st annual meeting of the New Clinical Drug Evaluation Unit of the National Institute of Mental Health, Phoenix, AZ, June 2000

Endicott J, Nee J, Harrison W, et al: Quality of Life Enjoyment and Satisfaction Questionnaire: a new measure. Psychopharmacol Bull 29:321–326, 1993

Fawcett J, Scheftner WA, Fogg L, et al: Time-related predictors of suicide in major affective disorder. Am J Psychiatry 147:1189–1194, 1990

Gastfriend DR, Rosenbaum JF: Adjunctive buspirone in benzodiazepine treatment of four patients with panic disorder. Am J Psychiatry 146:914–916, 1989

Gloger S, Grunhaus L, Gladic D, et al: Panic attacks and agoraphobia: low dose clomipramine treatment. J Clin Psychopharmacol 9:28–32, 1989

Gorman JM, Kent JM, Sullivan GM, et al: Neuroanatomical hypothesis of panic disorder, revised. Am J Psychiatry 157:493–505, 2000

Grove G, Coplan JD, Hollander E: The neuroanatomy of 5-HT dysregulation and panic disorder. J Neuropsychiatry Clin Neurosci 9:198–207, 1997

Herman JB, Rosenbaum JF, Brotman AW: The alprazolam to clonazepam switch for the treatment of panic disorder. J Clin Psychopharmacol 7:175–178, 1987

Hirschmann S, Dannon PN, Iancu I, et al: Pindolol augmentation in patients with treatment-resistant panic disorder: a double-blind, placebo-controlled trial. J Clin Psychopharmacol 20:556–559, 2000

Katon W, Vitaliano PP, Russo J, et al: Panic disorder: epidemiology in primary care. J Fam Pract 23:233–239, 1986

Kawachi I, Sparrow D, Vokonas PS, et al: Decreased heart rate variability in men with phobic anxiety (data from the Normative Aging Study). Am J Cardiol 75:882–885, 1995

Kawachi I, Sparrow D, Vokonas PS, et al: Symptoms of anxiety and risk of coronary heart disease. The Normative Aging Study. Circulation 90:2225–2229, 1994

Kessler RC, McGonagle KA, Zhao S, et al: Lifetime and 12-month prevalence of DSM-III-R psychiatric disorders in the United States: results from the National Comorbidity Survey. Arch Gen Psychiatry 51:8–19, 1994

Klein DF: Anxiety reconceptualized. Compr Psychiatry 21:411–427, 1980

Klein DF: False suffocation alarms, spontaneous panics, and related conditions: an integrative hypothesis. Arch Gen Psychiatry 50:306–317, 1993

Klein DF, Fink M: Psychiatric reaction patterns to imipramine. Am J Psychiatry 119:432–438, 1962

Klosko JS, Barlow DH, Tassinari R, et al: A comparison of alprazolam and behavior therapy in treatment of panic disorder: correction. J Consult Clin Psychol 63:830, 1995

Kruger MB, Dahl AA: The efficacy and safety of moclobemide compared to clomipramine in the treatment of panic disorder. Eur Arch Psychiatry Clin Neurosci 249 (suppl 1):S19–S24, 1999

LaBar KS, Gatenby JC, Gore JC, et al: Human amygdala activation during conditioned fear acquisition and extinction: a mixed-trial fMRI study. Neuron 20:937–945, 1998

LeDoux JE: Brain mechanisms of emotion and emotional learning. Curr Opin Neurobiol 2:191–197, 1992

Lydiard RB, Ballenger JC: Antidepressants in panic disorder and agoraphobia. J Affect Disord 13:153–168, 1987

Lydiard RB, Steiner M, Burnham D, et al: Efficacy studies of paroxetine in panic disorder. Psychopharmacol Bull 34: 175–182, 1998

Manfro GG, Otto MW, McArdle ET, et al: Relationship of antecedent stressful life events to childhood and family history of anxiety and the course of panic disorder. J Affect Disord 41:135–139, 1996

Mavissakalian M: Combined behavioral therapy and pharmacotherapy of agoraphobia. J Psychiatr Res 27 (suppl 1):179–191, 1993

Mavissakalian M, Perel JM: Protective effects of imipramine maintenance treatment in panic disorder with agoraphobia. Am J Psychiatry 149:1053–1057, 1992

Michelson D, Pollack M, Lydiard RB, et al: Continuing treatment of panic disorder after acute response: randomised, placebo-controlled trial with fluoxetine. The Fluoxetine Panic Disorder Study Group. Br J Psychiatry 174:213–218, 1999

Milrod B, Busch F, Leon AC, et al: A pilot open trial of brief psychodynamic psychotherapy for panic disorder. J Psychother Pract Res 10:239–245, 2001

Modigh K, Westbert P, Eriksson E: Superiority of clomipramine over imipramine in the treatment of panic disorder: a placebo-controlled trial. J Clin Psychopharmacol 12:251–261, 1992

Noyes R Jr., Burrows GD, Reich JH, et al: Diazepam versus alprazolam for the treatment of panic disorder. J Clin Psychiatry 57:349–355, 1996

Nutt DJ, Glue P, Lawson C, et al: Flumazenil provocation of panic attacks. Evidence for altered benzodiazepine receptor sensitivity in panic disorder. Arch Gen Psychiatry 47:917–925, 1990

Ontiveros A, Fontaine R: Sodium valproate and clonazepam for treatment-resistant panic disorder. J Psychiatry Neurosci 17:78–80, 1992

Otto MW, Pollack MH, Sachs GS, et al: Alcohol dependence in panic disorder patients. J Psychiatr Res 26:29–38, 1992a

Otto MW, Pollack MH, Meltzer-Brody S, et al: Cognitive-behavioral therapy for benzodiazepine discontinuation in panic disorder patients. Psychopharmacol Bull 28:123–130, 1992b

Otto MW, Pollack MH, Sabatino SA: Maintenance and remission following cognitive behavior therapy for panic disorder: possible deleterious effects of concurrent medication treatment. Behav Ther 27:473–482, 1996

Otto MW, Pollack MH, Sachs GS, et al: Discontinuation of benzodiazepine treatment: efficacy of cognitive-behavioral therapy for patients with panic disorder. Am J Psychiatry 150:1485–1490, 1993

Pande AC, Pollack MH, Crockatt J, et al: Placebo-controlled study of gabapentin treatment of panic disorder. J Clin Psychopharmacol 20:467–471, 2000

Papp LA, Coplan JD, Martinez JM, et al: Efficacy of open-label nefazodone treatment in patients with panic disorder. J Clin Psychopharmacol 20:544–546, 2000

Pollack MH, Marzol PC: Panic: course, complications and treatment of panic disorder. J Psychopharmacol 14 (2 suppl 1):S25–S30, 2000

Pollack MH, Otto MW: Long-term course and outcome of panic disorder. J Clin Psychiatry 58 (suppl 2):57–60, 1997

Pollack MH, Otto MW, Majcher D, et al: Relationship of childhood anxiety to adult panic disorder: correlates and influence on course. Am J Psychiatry 153:376–381, 1996a

Pollack MH, Worthington JJ 3rd, Otto MW, et al: Venlafaxine for panic disorder: results from a double-blind, placebo-controlled study. Psychopharmacol Bull 32:667–670, 1996b

Pollack MH, Matthews J, Scott EL: Gabapentin as a potential treatment for anxiety disorders. Am J Psychiatry 155:992–993, 1998

Rapaport MH, Wolkow R, Rubin A, et al: Sertraline treatment of panic disorder: results of a long-term study. Acta Psychiatr Scand 104:289–298, 2001

Redmond DE Jr, Huang YH, Snyder DR, et al: Behavioral effects of stimulation of the nucleus locus coeruleus in the stump-tailed monkey *Macaca arctoides*. Brain Res 116:502–510, 1976

Rickels K, Schweizer E, Case WG, et al: Long-term therapeutic use of benzodiazepines: effects of abrupt discontinuation. Arch Gen Psychiatry 47:899–907, 1990

Rimon R, Lepola U, Jolkkonen J, et al: Cerebrospinal fluid gamma-aminobutyric acid in patients with panic disorder. Biol Psychiatry 38:737–741, 1995

Sartorius N, Ustun TB, Costa e Silva JA, et al: An international study of psychological problems in primary care: preliminary report from the World Health Organization Collaborative Project on "Psychological Problems in General Health Care."s Arch Gen Psychiatry 50:819–824, 1993

Scott EL, Pollack MH, Otto MW, et al: Clinician response to treatment refractory panic disorder: a survey of psychiatrists. J Nerv Ment Dis 187:755–757, 1999

Shear MK, Maser JD: Standardized assessment for panic disorder research. Arch Gen Psychiatry 51:346–354, 1994

Shear MK, Brown TA, Barlow DH, et al: Multicenter collaborative panic disorder severity scale. Am J Psychiatry 154:1571–1575, 1997

Shear MK, Houck P, Greeno C, et al: Emotion-focused psychotherapy for patients with panic disorder. Am J Psychiatry 158:1993–1998, 2001

Sheehan DV: The Anxiety Disease. New York, Charles Scribner's Sons, 1983

Sheehan DV, Harnett-Sheehan K: The role of SSRIs in panic disorder. J Clin Psychiatry 57 (suppl 10):51–58, 1996

Sheehan DV, Davidson J, Manschreck T, et al: Lack of efficacy of a new antidepressant (bupropion) in the treatment of panic disorder with phobias. J Clin Psychopharmacol 3:28–31, 1983

Sheehan DV, Raj AB, Harnett-Sheehan K, et al: The relative efficacy of high-dose buspirone and alprazolam in the treatment of panic disorder: a double-blind placebo-controlled study. Acta Psychiatr Scand 88:1–11, 1993

Shekhar A, Keim SR, Simon JR, et al: Dorsomedial hypothalamic GABA dysfunction produces physiological arousal following sodium lactate infusions. Pharmacol Biochem Behav 55:249–256, 1996

Simon GE, VonKorff M: Somatization and psychiatric disorders in the NIMH Epidemiologic Catchment Area study. Am J Psychiatry 148:1494–1500, 1991

Simon NM, Pollack M: Treatment-refractory panic disorder. Psychiatr Clin North Am 6:115–140, 1999

Simon NM, Safren SA, Otto MW, et al: Longitudinal outcome with pharmacotherapy in a naturalistic study of panic disorder. J Affect Disord 69:201–208, 2002

Telch MJ, Lucas RA, Schmidt NB, et al: Group cognitive-behavioral treatment of panic disorder. Behav Res Ther 31:279–287, 1993

Tesar GE, Rosenbaum JF, Pollack MH, et al: Double-blind, placebo-controlled comparison of clonazepam and alprazolam for panic disorder. J Clin Psychiatry 52:69–76, 1991

Tiffon L, Coplan JD, Papp LA, et al: Augmentation strategies with tricyclic or fluoxetine treatment in seven partially responsive panic disorder patients. J Clin Psychiatry 55:66–69, 1994

Tucker P, Adamson P, Miranda R Jr, et al: Paroxetine increases heart rate variability in panic disorder. J Clin Psychopharmacol 17:370–376, 1997

Uhde TW, Stein MB, Post RM, et al: Lack of efficacy of carbamazepine in the treatment of panic disorder. Am J Psychiatry 145:1104–1109, 1988

Uhlenhuth EH: Treatment strategies in panic disorder: recommendations of an expert panel. Paper presented at the World Regional Congress of Biological Psychiatry, São Paulo, Brazil, April 1998

van Vliet IM, den Boer JA, Westenberg HG, et al: A double-blind comparative study of brofaromine and fluvoxamine in outpatients with panic disorder. J Clin Psychopharmacol 16:299–306, 1996

Ware JE Jr, Sherbourne CD: The MOS 36-item short-form health survey (SF-36), I: conceptual framework and item selection. Med Care 30:473–483, 1992

Weissman MM, Klerman GL, Markowitz JS, et al: Suicidal ideation and suicide attempts in panic disorder and attacks. N Engl J Med 321:1209–1214, 1989

Wilborg IM, Dahl AA: Does brief dynamic psychotherapy reduce the relapse rate of panic disorder? Arch Gen Psychiatry 53:689–694, 1996

Woodman CL, Noyes R: Panic disorder: treatment with valproate. J Clin Psychiatry 55:134–136, 1994

3

Specific Phobia

Bavanisha Vythilingum, M.B.

Dan J. Stein, M.D., Ph.D.

Phenomenology

Symptoms

Specific phobia is defined as the circumscribed fear of an object or situation and is characterized by marked and persistent fear of the object or situation, together with a desire to avoid it. As objects of phobias are generally those things that evoke fear and distaste in the general population, many people with this disorder have viewed it as "normal." DSM-IV-TR (American Psychiatric Association 2000) emphasizes, however, the disability associated with specific phobia, with a diagnosis requiring functional impairment and/or marked distress (Table 3–1).

The most striking difference between DSM-IV-TR and DSM-III-R criteria (American Psychiatric Association 1987) is the name change from *simple phobia* to *specific phobia*. The phobias have tended to be erroneously perceived as less serious forms of psychiatric disorder, and the renaming of the condition

Table 3–1.   DSM-IV-TR diagnostic criteria for specific phobia

A. Marked and persistent fear that is excessive or unreasonable, cued by the presence or anticipation of a specific object or situation (e.g., flying, heights, animals, receiving an injection, seeing blood).

B. Exposure to the phobic stimulus almost invariably provokes an immediate anxiety response, which may take the form of a situationally bound or situationally predisposed panic attack.   **Note:** In children, the anxiety may be expressed by crying, tantrums, freezing, or clinging.

C. The person recognizes that the fear is excessive or unreasonable.   **Note:** In children, this feature may be absent.

D. The phobic situation(s) is avoided or else is endured with intense anxiety or distress.

E. The avoidance, anxious anticipation, or distress in the feared situation(s) interferes significantly with the person's normal routine, occupational (or academic) functioning, or social activities or relationships, or there is marked distress about having the phobia.

F. In individuals under age 18 years, the duration is at least 6 months.

G. The anxiety, panic attacks, or phobic avoidance associated with the specific object or situation are not better accounted for by another mental disorder, such as obsessive-compulsive disorder (e.g., fear of dirt in someone with an obsession about contamination), posttraumatic stress disorder (e.g., avoidance of stimuli associated with a severe stressor), separation anxiety disorder (e.g., avoidance of school), social phobia (e.g., avoidance of social situations because of fear of embarrassment), panic disorder with agoraphobia, or agoraphobia without history of panic disorder.

Specify type:

> **Animal Type**
> **Natural Environment Type** (e.g., heights, storms, water)
> **Blood-Injection-Injury Type**
> **Situational Type** (e.g., airplanes, elevators, enclosed places)
> **Other Type** (e.g., fear of choking, vomiting, or contracting an illness; in children, fear of loud sounds or costumed characters)

as specific phobia removes the misleading sense of a benign disorder that is associated with the term *simple* (Marks 1987). It also brings DSM-IV-TR in line with ICD-10 (*International Statistical Classification of Diseases and Related Health Problems*, 10th Revision) (World Health Organization 1992).

DSM-IV-TR criteria for specific phobia also explicitly allow for the occurrence of panic attacks in response to the feared stimulus. In contrast,

DSM-III-R criteria, although not excluding the possibility of panic attacks, did not mention them, possibly allowing some diagnostic confusion.

Associated Features

Comorbidity in specific phobia is very common, with rates of up to 65% (Starcevic and Bogojevic 1997). The most important predictor of comorbidity is number of fears, irrespective of type and/or severity (Curtis et al. 1998). Other anxiety disorders are the most frequent comorbid Axis I disorders (Goisman et al. 1998), with posttraumatic stress disorder (Goisman et al. 1998) and social phobia (Turner et al. 1991) being the most prevalent. Interestingly, specific phobia may be unique in predicting the persistence of social phobia. Uncomplicated panic disorder, however, was found to be associated with a decreased incidence of specific phobia (Goisman et al. 1998).

Substance use disorders are also common; approximately one-tenth of patients with specific phobia have hazardous alcohol use (Sareen et al. 2001). Specific phobia in itself may constitute an independent risk factor for alcohol abuse; a significant association was found between specific phobia and the development of alcohol abuse (Sareen et al. 2001). Furthermore, children of alcoholics were shown to have an increased prevalence of specific phobia as compared with a control group (Mathew et al. 1993).

Comorbid depression is also common (Curtis et al. 1998), particularly in adolescents. One-third of adolescents with a primary diagnosis of specific phobia have comorbid depression (Essau et al. 2000). Indeed, specific phobia, particularly if comorbid depression is present, is a risk factor for suicidal behavior. Thus, a study of patients who attempted suicide found that after depression, specific phobia was the second most common primary diagnosis (Rudd et al. 1993).

A few small studies suggest that gender and ethnicity may influence patterns of comorbidity in specific phobia. Fava et al. (1996) found that depressed women were more likely than depressed men to have comorbid specific phobia. In another small study, Ziedonis et al. (1994) found that among cocaine addicts, woman were more likely than men and African Americans were more likely than whites to have specific phobia. However, available data on this issue are limited, and more work is needed to clarify whether ethnicity and gender do in fact influence comorbidity.

The relationship between specific phobia and personality disorders is less well documented than Axis I comorbidity. Sanderson et al. (1994) found that personality disorders occurred infrequently with specific phobia, in only 12% of subjects. The relationship between the type of personality disorder and specific phobia is also unclear. Alnaes and Torgersen (1988) found an association between Cluster B but not Cluster C disorders and specific phobia. However, Okasha et al. (1996) found an association between avoidant personality disorder and specific phobia, whereas Nestadt et al. (1992) found that higher scores on measures of compulsive personality were associated with an increased risk for specific phobia.

Epidemiology

Specific phobia is one of the most common psychiatric disorders, with prevalence rates varying from 4.7% (Hwu et al. 1989) to 11.3% (Kessler et al. 1994). This wide variation has been attributed to difficulties in defining when a fear becomes a phobia. Many phobia-inducing stimuli (such as blood, snakes, and heights) evoke fear in most people, and the decision as to when this becomes unreasonable or excessive depends to a degree on the investigators' judgment (and perhaps own fears). Nevertheless, two of the largest epidemiological studies, the Epidemiologic Catchment Area (ECA) study (Eaton and Kessler 1991) and the National Comorbidity Survey (NCS) (Magee et al. 1996) found remarkably similar rates (11.25% and 11.3%, respectively) despite using different structured interviews (Diagnostic Interview Schedule vs. Composite International Diagnostic Interview) and different diagnostic criteria (DSM-III vs. DSM-III-R). This consistency suggests that specific phobia indeed occurs much more commonly than its prevalence in clinical settings would suggest.

Numerous studies have confirmed that specific phobia is more common in women than in men, with prevalence rates ranging from 6% to 26.5% in women, as compared with only 2.3% to 12.4% in men (Fredrikson et al. 1996). This sex-related difference may reflect the more frequent occurrence of role modeling in women (Fredrikson et al. 1996), thus facilitating social transmission of fears and phobias. Essau et al. (2000) found a 3.5% lifetime prevalence for specific phobia in adolescents, with more girls than boys meeting diagnostic criteria, whereas a study of children ages 4–12 years found a prevalence of 17.6% (Muris and Merckelbach 2000). The ECA study (Boyd et al. 1990) found increased prevalence of specific phobia with younger age.

In the ECA study (Eaton and Kessler 1991), clear ethnic differences were found, with prevalences in black individuals being consistently higher than in whites or Hispanics. Studies in Taiwan (Hwu et al. 1989) and Korea (Lee et al. 1990) found prevalences of 3.6% and 2.7%, respectively, which is rather lower than the 11.25% reported in the ECA study (Eaton and Kessler 1991). Whether this difference is related to ethnicity per se, however, is not clear, and it may represent different thresholds for considering a fear unreasonable. Low socioeconomic status was found to be a risk factor for increased prevalence of specific phobia in the ECA study (Boyd et al. 1990).

Assessment

Patients with specific phobia deserve a comprehensive psychiatric evaluation that focuses not only the phobic symptoms but also on their functional consequences and on determining whether comorbid disorders are present. In addition, the particular phobias present should be explored in detail. DSM-IV-TR, for example, classifies phobias into four subtypes: animal, situational, natural environment, blood/injection/injury (BII), and animal (Table 3–1). Situational phobias are the most common, animal phobias the least common. In this section, we provide relevant information about each of these subtypes.

Situational phobias include phobias such as acrophobia (fear of heights) and claustrophobia (fear of enclosed spaces). Situational phobias tend to have a later age at onset relative to other phobias (Himle et al. 1991), with a mean age at onset in the 20s. There is some evidence to suggest that unexpected panic attacks may be more prevalent with this type of phobia (Ehlers 1995). Patients with situational phobia also report a higher incidence of spontaneous phobia onset than other phobia patients (Himle et al. 1991). It has been postulated that situational phobias may be related to panic disorder and agoraphobia (Himle et al. 1989); however, not all studies have confirmed this (Antony et al. 1997a).

Natural environment phobias include fears of such things as storms and water. Natural environment phobias as a category have not been well studied, and controversy exists over whether this is best conceptualized as a separate category or as a subtype of situational phobias. There is also controversy over which phobias fall into this category; for example, some authors consider heights to fall into this category.

BII phobias have a prevalence of approximately 3%–5% (Bienvenu and Eaton 1998) in the general population. These phobias are distinct from the other phobias in that they are characterized by a biphasic physiological reaction. When confronted by their phobia stimulus, phobic patients usually show increases in heart rate, blood pressure, and skin conductance, which gradually return to normal on prolonged exposure (Marks 1987). However, in patients with BII phobias, this elevation in heart rate and blood pressure is transient and is followed by a rapid drop to below baseline levels, often resulting in fainting (Thyer et al. 1985). BII phobias usually start in childhood or adolescence; onset in adulthood is rare (Himle et al. 1989). BII phobias tend to run in families, with both modeling and genetic factors being proposed as etiological contributors. However, the higher concordance between monozygotic than dizygotic twins (0.59 vs. 0.08) suggests a genetic component in their acquisition.

Animal phobias, like BII phobias, tend to begin earlier than other subtypes, with a mean age at onset of 7 years (Himle et al. 1989; Ost 1992). Animal phobias appear to be more common in women, with Fredrikson et al. (1996) reporting a rate of 12.1% in women, compared with only 3.3% in men. Panic attacks may be more common in this type of phobia, as well as more predictable (Antony et al. 1997a).

Empirical data on the validity of these subtypes vary, with evidence being strongest for BII phobia and least strong for natural environment and situational phobias. Fredrikson et al. (1996), in a factor analysis of adults' fear ratings of potentially phobogenic objects and situations, showed that specific phobia symptoms clustered around three factors: animal, BII, and a factor combining natural environment and situational phobias. A confirmatory factor analysis in children (Muris et al. 1999b) replicated these findings. Antony et al. (1997a) suggested that certain natural environment phobias, such as heights, may best be classified as a type of situational phobia and that in view of the difficulty in classifying certain types of phobias (e.g., whether bridge phobia is a situational or a natural environment phobia), it may be better to eliminate the classification altogether and simply name the specific phobia.

Pathogenesis

Basic Physiology and Anatomy of Fear

Emotions can be grouped into two categories on the basis of motivational organization: pleasant (associated with appetitive drives) and unpleasant (associated with defensive reactions). It is the defensive reactions that produce the emotional and physiological components associated with fear and anxiety (Konorski 1967).

Several structures within the brain participate in the production of anxiety, but it is the amygdala, an almond-shaped structure deep within the temporal lobe, that is key in both the experience of and the acquisition of fear. The amygdala receives input through its lateral and basolateral nucleus, and output is via the central nucleus. From the central nucleus, wide projections mediate different aspects of fear. These can be divided into two broad output classes: freezing responses and defensive action (fight/flight response; Penick et al. 1994).

When a stimulus is paired with a threat, on subsequent exposure to the stimulus an increased startle response is elicited. This has been termed *fear-potentiated startle* (Brown et al. 1951). The central nucleus of the amygdala plays a key role in this; lesioning of the nucleus has been shown to block the startle response in previously sensitized animals (Hitchcock and Davis 1986). Other structures, including the hippocampus, may play a role in more defensive responses, including avoidance of feared stimuli.

Corticotropin-releasing hormone (CRH) has an enhancing anxiogenic effect on the startle response (Liang et al. 1992). The primary receptors that mediate this effect are in the bed nucleus of stria terminalis (an area near to but distinct from the amygdala). CRH enhancement is also noted to be long-lasting (Lang et al. 2000). It is possible that the bed nucleus of the stria terminalis mediates anxiety (a long-lasting emotion), whereas the amygdala mediates fear (which is more short-lived). Neurons in the central nucleus of the amygdala are CRH releasing and project to the bed nucleus (Sakanaka et al. 1986). Thus, activation of the amygdala may lead to long-term activation of the bed nucleus because of the action of CRH, with a prolonged anxiogenic effect.

Application to Specific Phobia

Prey animals have been shown to detect threat quickly (Dawkins and Krebs 1979). It seems reasonable to suggest that humans can react similarly, reacting quickly to signs of danger even if these are brief or unclear. Seligman (1971) proposed that humans have a biological preparedness to acquire certain fears; on the basis of evolutionarily acquired cues, certain fears would be acquired more rapidly and with less exposure. Lang (1985) further suggested that the amygdala network was hyperactive in specific phobia, with rapid activation after even degraded stimuli.

Specific phobia may be postulated to be an abnormal activation of the fear network, with the limited range of phobias occurring as a result of evolutionarily relevant "prepared fears." Symptoms may be accounted for by amygdala activation and differential activation of the various output pathways. This could, for example, explain low blood pressure and fainting in BII phobia, where the output pathway to the dorsomedial nucleus of the vagus may be preferentially activated.

A growing body of clinical data provides evidence for involvement of such a fear network in specific phobia. Perhaps most persuasively, positron emission tomography studies of patients with specific phobia show increased blood flow to the paralimbic cortex and activation of neuronal pathways in the amygdala, thalamus, and striatum (Wik et al. 1996).

Carbon dioxide challenge studies have also been used to explore the fear network in specific phobia but have shown mixed results. In a study using 35% carbon dioxide, subjects with situational but not animal phobia showed increased anxiety as compared with control subjects (Verburg et al. 1994), suggesting a possible relationship between situational phobia and panic disorder. However, in a second study (this time using 5.5% carbon dioxide), patients with specific phobia had responses that fell between those of the patients with panic disorder and the control subjects (Antony et al. 1997b). On the few measures in which specific phobia subgroups differed from each other, those with situational and natural environment phobia showed the greatest response. It is possible that specific phobia may represent more limited activation of the fear network as compared with more general activation in panic disorder.

Etiological Models

Abnormal activation of the fear network has been proposed as important in mediating specific phobia, but why does such activation occur? Two etiological models—modified conditioning and nonassociative—have been proposed.

Modified Conditioning Model

Modified conditioning is similar to classical conditioning but, in an effort to explain why in many patients no conditioning event is reported, postulates that the conditioning event is forgotten. How could a conditioning event be forgotten but emotional memory retained? There are two pathways for the acquisition of fear—a subcortical pathway that is rapid, passing directly from the thalamus to the amygdala, and a cortical pathway that is slower but has access to the hippocampus and is involved in the formation of explicit memories (Tillier et al. 1997).

It is postulated either that there is maturational lag in the cortical pathway, so that emotional but not explicit memory is encoded (Jacobs and Nadel 1985), or that with stress, the release of CRH and cortisol impairs hippocampal function (Bremner et al. 1995) but does not impair or possibly even enhances amygdala function (McGaugh et al. 1993). In either scenario, emotional memories are formed without an accompanying explicit memory.

However, several shortcomings exist with this model (Rachman et al. 1987). First, phobias have been shown to cluster into distinct categories, whereas conditioning proposes that all stimuli can become feared. Seligman's (1971) preparedness theory of fear acquisition (in which humans are biologically prepared to develop certain fears as a result of evolutionary pressures) may, however, be used to supplement the model to address this. Second, many patients experience aversive conditioning but do not develop phobias, suggesting that additional factors are important. Conversely, there is evidence attesting to indirect and vicarious modes of onset for phobias (Rachman et al. 1987).

Nonassociative Models

Nonassociative models postulate that certain intrinsic fears are a normal part of development and that specific phobias represent the failure of habituation of these intrinsic fears (Menzies and Clarke 1995). For example, all infants experience the fear of height as a natural developmental phase in the period before they begin to walk. In visual cliff experiments (Gibson and Walk 1960), where a transparent board is placed over a patterned fabric, which then falls away, producing the illusion of a cliff, infants refuse to cross. However, as they mature and begin to walk, they begin to lose this fear. It is possible that nonhabituation may lead to the development of acrophobia. Nonhabituation has been postulated to occur through failure of learning from experience or failure of safe exposure (Menzies and Clarke 1995).

Empirical evidence for a nonassociative model is so far limited. Twin studies show moderate heritability (0.3–0.4) of specific phobias, which is in keeping with this model (Kendler et al. 1992). In a recent study, Kendler et al. (2002) examined the mode of acquisition of fears in twins. They proposed that if the development of specific phobias was related to traumatic exposure (as with modified conditioning), the degree of environmental stress associated with fear onset would correlate inversely with endogenous liability to phobia proneness. That is, in those twins who could remember a trauma associated with the onset of fear, rates of phobias should be lower in their co-twin, as compared with those twins who could not remember an event. The risk of phobias, however, was not found to be elevated in co-twins of twins with no memory of the mode of acquisition of the fear, and the risk of phobias was not decreased in co-twins of twins with severe trauma to the self. Furthermore, no significant relationship was found in the phobic twins between levels of neuroticism and mode of acquisition of fear. The authors concluded that their data were not compatible with a conditioning/learning theory but rather suggested that vulnerability to phobias is largely innate.

The Role of Disgust

Disgust is an emotional response to threat of disease transmission or contamination (Rozin and Fallon 1987). Disgust may play a particular role in the genesis of specific phobia—particularly small-animal phobias. Matchett and Davey (1991) found a positive association between measures of disgust and scores on the animal section of the Fear Survey Schedule. These findings have since been replicated.

Correlation between parental and offspring disgust scores have also been found (Davey et al. 1993), and parental disgust sensitivity is a good predictor of offsprings' small-animal fears. Girls with spider phobia were found to have higher levels of disgust and felt spiders to be more disgusting than control subjects did. After treatment, reduction in fear was paralleled by a decline in the disgust-evoking status of spiders (de Jong et al. 1997).

It is possible that the contribution of disgust to phobias is subtype specific, being restricted to small-animal and BII phobias. Fainting in BII may be mediated by the vagal mechanism of disgust (Levenson 1992). Speculatively, patients with animal phobia may not faint because sympathetic activation overrides parasympathetic activation. Some empirical data exist to support this—in BII, disgust rather than fear is experienced on exposure to pictorial stimuli, whereas in spider phobia, both fear and disgust are experienced (Tolin et al. 1997).

However, disgust may underlie a broad range of anxiety disorders (Phillips et al. 1998). In normal schoolchildren, for example, disgust sensitivity correlated positively with a number of anxiety disorders, and associations were also found between disgust sensitivity and trait anxiety (Muris et al. 1999a). However, when disgust sensitivity scores were controlled for trait anxiety, then correlations between disgust and anxiety disorders disappeared, except in specific phobias, where a modest correlation remained. Thus, disgust sensitivity in most anxiety disorders may not be independent of trait anxiety, but in specific phobia it may represent an independent vulnerability factor.

Pharmacotherapy

Pharmacotherapy for phobias is less well studied than psychotherapy. However, several reports suggest that medication may be a useful treatment, alone or in combination with psychotherapy.

An early study found that the monoamine oxidase inhibitor phenelzine was effective in patients with a range of different phobias, including social phobia, agoraphobia, and specific phobias. However, these agents are now rarely used in view of the associated inconvenience and adverse events. The tricyclic antidepressant imipramine has also been used in the treatment of specific phobia, but comparisons with placebo have not shown a significant advantage (Zitrin et al. 1983).

There is also some evidence that selective serotonin reuptake inhibitors (SSRIs) are effective in specific phobia. There have been several case studies reporting efficacy in the treatment of specific phobias (Abene and Hamilton 1998), and one small double-blind study (Benjamin et al. 2000) found paroxetine to be superior to placebo. SSRIs may be particularly useful in settings where psychotherapy is not available or where comorbid conditions that respond to these agents also exist. Figure 3–1 presents a treatment algorithm.

Benzodiazepines may be useful where immediate intervention is needed, but their risk–benefit ratio suggests that they should not be relied on for long-term treatment. Similarly, data on β-blockers for conditions such as flight phobia are mixed (Campos et al. 1984).

Psychotherapy

Psychotherapy has been the mainstay of treatment for specific phobias. Psychotherapies can be divided on a theoretical basis into behavioral and cogni-

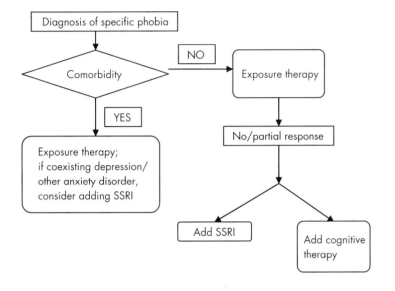

Figure 3–1.   Algorithm for treatment of specific phobia.
SSRI = selective serotonin reuptake inhibitor.

tive approaches. In practice, a combination of these approaches is often used. However, for the purposes of this chapter, we discuss each approach individually and thereafter examine combination therapy.

Behavioral Approaches

Behavioral approaches are based on behavioral theories of phobias, which, as discussed earlier, emphasize learning experiences or lack of habituation to specific situations. Behavioral approaches thus concentrate on "unlearning" or "correcting faulty learning." The mainstay of behavioral intervention for specific phobia is exposure therapy. Exposure therapy consists of gradual exposure to the feared stimulus until extinction of the fear response occurs. Exposure therapy can be conducted in various ways (Craske and Rowe 1997), including

1. Imaginal versus in vivo
2. Graded versus intense (sometimes known as *flooding*)

3. Therapist-aided versus self-directed
4. Continuation of exposure until anxiety subsides versus termination at point of heightened anxiety, followed by reexposure when anxiety has subsided

Relaxation techniques, including progressive relaxation training and breathing methods, are also used, usually in conjunction with exposure therapy.

We have mentioned that behavioral therapy involves the "unlearning" of the fear, but by what mechanisms does this occur? Several theories have been proposed to explain this process.

Habituation refers to the reduction in response strength with repeated presentations of the stimulus. Groves and Thompson (1970) suggested that observed behavior is a result of the summation of two processes—sensitization (increasing responsiveness with repeated presentation of the stimuli) and habituation. There is some empirical support for the role of habituation in exposure therapy. Patients with specific phobia who exhibit greater physiological habituation have a better overall outcome (Marshall 1988). Furthermore, several independent variables, including level of arousal, dependent drugs, and rate and complexity of stimulation, affect both habituation and fear reduction during exposure in the same way (Rachman et al. 1987).

However, there are limitations to habituation as a proposed sole mechanism for the efficacy of behavior therapy. Fears persist despite repeated stimulus presentations. Furthermore, flooding is effective therapy for phobias, yet habituation is impeded by intense stimuli (Rachman et al. 1987). In addition, exposure therapy has long-term effects, whereas habituation is a transient process that naturally dishabituates in the absence of continued stimulus exposure.

Extinction is another mechanism proposed for the efficacy of behavior therapy. It refers to a decreasing fearful response generated through repeated encounters with a feared stimulus without aversive consequences. A nonfearful pairing is thus generated. Bouton (2002) has postulated that during extinction, the original excitatory meaning of the feared stimulus is not erased but instead an additional inhibitory meaning is learned. Context is important in determining which memory is retrieved (e.g., a snake in a cage may not be viewed as dangerous, whereas one in the wild is). Return of fear after therapy is thus viewed as a contextual retrieval of the excitatory meaning. The postulates of Bouton have therapeutic implications—lengthy exposure in a variety of contexts and naturalistic settings may be necessary for a complete response.

Another mechanism proposed for exposure therapy is an *alteration in the predictive accuracy* of the phobic patient. Typically, patients with specific phobia overestimate the level of threat. By repeated exposure without adverse consequences, individuals learn to predict consequences more accurately and thus to have diminished anxiety (Rachman et al. 1987). However, this suggestion, too, has not yet been empirically confirmed (van den Hout et al. 1997)

There is growing interest in the neurobiology of extinction. Early work suggested release of endorphins in response to fear may promote extinction by reinforcing approach behavior or reducing the aversiveness of the exposure. Some empirical evidence exists to support this: administration of naloxone, an opioid antagonist, impeded imaginal exposure significantly more than saline placebos (Egan et al. 1988). More recent work has emphasized the role of GABA (γ-aminobutyric acid) in inhibiting brain areas involved in fear learning, and of glutamate in mediating the relevant neuronal plasticity (Davis and Myers 2002).

Cognitive Approaches

The cognitive approach has as its basis the recognition of characteristic distortions in thinking in anxious patients that reflect perceptions of harm or danger. Anxious patients are more likely to perceive neutral or ambiguous stimuli as threatening. In specific phobia, the phobic stimulus is thus perceived as dangerous (Di Nardo et al. 1988).

Cognitive-based therapies focus on correcting underlying cognitive distortions through conscious reasoning. In specific phobia, reductions in negative cognitions have been correlated with reduction in fear and, similarly, return of fear has been correlated with return of negative cognitions (Shafran et al. 1993). However, whether cognitive change is causal in fear reduction or instead follows it has not yet been empirically demonstrated (Rachman et al. 1987).

Efficacy of Behavioral and Cognitive Treatments

Exposure therapy has consistently been found effective in the treatment of specific phobia, with imaginal procedures less effective than in vivo exposure (Barlow et al. 1969; Crowe et al. 1972; Mathews 1987). Although early literature suggested that specific phobias were not treatable via cognitive therapy, more recent studies have shown efficacy for this intervention (Booth and Rachman 1992; de Jongh et al. 1995).

Studies of combined exposure and cognitive therapy have shown mixed results. Emmelkamp and Felten (1985) found some superiority for combined treatment over exposure therapy alone in the treatment of patients with acrophobia. In patients with fear of flying, exposure combined with cognitive restructuring was more effective than exposure therapy alone (Ost et al. 1997). However, in a study of patients with dental phobia, no difference in outcome was observed between combined treatment and behavioral treatment alone (Getka and Glass 1992).

Conclusion

Specific phobia is a disorder that has for many years been viewed as mild and perhaps trivial. However, there is now growing recognition of the extent of associated distress and impairment. Advances have been made in our understanding both of why specific phobia occurs and how it can be treated. Although exposure therapy remains the mainstay of treatment for specific phobia, pharmacotherapy also deserves consideration, particularly should comorbid mood and anxiety conditions exist.

References

Abene MV, Hamilton JD: Resolution of fear of flying with fluoxetine treatment. J Anxiety Disord 12:599–603, 1998

Alnaes R, Torgersen S: The relationship between DSM-III symptom disorders (Axis I) and personality disorders (Axis II) in an outpatient population. Acta Psychiatr Scand 78:485–492, 1988

American Psychiatric Association: Diagnostic and Statistical Manual of Mental Disorders, 3rd Edition, Revised. Washington, DC, American Psychiatric Association, 1987

American Psychiatric Association: Diagnostic and Statistical Manual of Mental Disorders, 4th Edition, Text Revision. Washington, DC, American Psychiatric Association, 2000

Antony MM, Brown TA, Barlow DH: Heterogeneity among specific phobia types in DSM-IV-TR. Behav Res Ther 35:1089–1100, 1997a

Antony MM, Brown TA, Barlow DH: Response to hyperventilation and 5.5% CO_2 inhalation of subjects with types of specific phobia, panic disorder, or no mental disorder. Am J Psychiatry 154:1089–1095, 1997b

Barlow DH, Leitenberg HM, Agras WS, et al: The transfer gap in systematic desensitization: an analogue study. Behav Res Ther 7:191–196, 1969

Benjamin J, Ben Zion IZ, Karbofsky E, et al: Double-blind placebo-controlled pilot study of paroxetine for specific phobia. Psychopharmacology (Berl) 149:194–196, 2000

Bienvenu OJ, Eaton WW: The epidemiology of blood-injection-injury phobia. Psychol Med 28:1129–1136, 1998

Booth R, Rachman S: The reduction of claustrophobia, I. Behav Res Ther 30:207–221, 1992

Bouton ME: Context, ambiguity, and unlearning: sources of relapse after behavioral extinction. Biol Psychiatry 52:976–986, 2002

Boyd JH, Rae DS, Thompson JW, et al: Phobia: prevalence and risk factors. Soc Psychiatry Psychiatr Epidemiol 25:314–323, 1990

Bremner JD, Krystal JH, Southwick SM, et al: Functional neuroanatomical correlates of the effects of stress on memory. J Trauma Stress 8:527–553, 1995

Brown JS, Kalish HI, Farber IE: Conditional fear as revealed by magnitude of startle response to an auditory stimulus. J Exp Psychol 41:317–328, 1951

Campos PE, Solyom L, Koelink A: The effects of timolol maleate on subjective and physiological components of air travel phobia. Can J Psychiatry 29:570–574, 1984

Craske MG, Rowe MK: A comparison of behavioral and cognitive treatments of phobias, in Phobias: A Handbook of Theory, Research and Treatment. Edited by Davey GC. New York, Wiley, 1997, pp 247–280

Crowe MJ, Marks IM, Agras WS, et al: Time-limited desensitization, implosion and shaping for phobic patients: a cross-over study. Behav Res Ther 10:667–685, 1972

Curtis GC, Magee WJ, Eaton WW, et al: Specific fears and phobias: epidemiology and classification. Br J Psychiatry 173:212–217, 1998

Davey GC, Forster L, Mayhew G: Familial resemblances in disgust sensitivity and animal phobias. Behav Res Ther 31:41–50, 1993

Davis M, Myers KM: The role of glutamate and gamma-aminobutyric acid in fear extinction: clinical implications for exposure therapy. Biol Psychiatry 52:998–1007, 2002

Dawkins R, Krebs JR: Arms races between and within species. Proc R Soc Lond B Biol Sci 205:489–511, 1979

de Jong PJ, Andrea H, Muris P: Spider phobia in children: disgust and fear before and after treatment. Behav Res Ther 35:559–562, 1997

de Jongh A, Muris P, ter Horst G, et al: One-session cognitive treatment of dental phobia: preparing dental phobics for treatment by restructuring negative cognitions. Behav Res Ther 33:947–954, 1995

Di Nardo PA, Guzy LT, Bak RM: Anxiety response patterns and etiological factors in dog-fearful and non-fearful subjects. Behav Res Ther 26:245–252, 1988

Eaton WW, Kessler LG: Panic and phobia, in Psychiatric Disorders in America: The Epidemiologic Catchment Area Study. Edited by Robins LN, Regier DA. New York, Free Press, 1991, pp 155–179

Egan KJ, Carr JE, Hunt DD, et al: Endogenous opiate system and systematic desensitization. J Consult Clin Psychol 56:287–291, 1988

Ehlers A: A 1-year prospective study of panic attacks: clinical course and factors associated with maintenance. J Abnorm Psychol 104:164–172, 1995

Emmelkamp PMG, Felten M: The process of exposure in vivo: cognitive and physiological changes during the treatment of acrophobia. Behav Res Ther 23:219–233, 1985

Essau CA, Conradt J, Petermann F: Frequency, comorbidity, and psychosocial impairment of specific phobia in adolescents. J Clin Child Psychol 29:221–231, 2000

Fava M, Abraham M, Alpert J, et al: Gender differences in Axis I comorbidity among depressed outpatients. J Affect Disord 38:129–133, 1996

Fredrikson M, Annas P, Fischer H, et al: Gender and age differences in the prevalence of specific fears and phobias. Behav Res Ther 34:33–39, 1996

Getka EJ, Glass CR: Behavioral and cognitive-behavioral approaches to the reduction of dental anxiety. Behavior Therapy 23:433–448, 1992

Gibson EJ, Walk RD: The "visual cliff." Scientific American 202:2–9, 1960

Goisman RM, Allsworth J, Rogers MP, et al: Simple phobia as a comorbid anxiety disorder. Depress Anxiety 7:105–112, 1998

Groves PM, Thompson RF: Habituation: a dual process theory. Psychol Rev 77:419–450, 1970

Himle JA, McPhee K, Cameron OG, et al: Simple phobia: evidence for heterogeneity. Psychiatry Res 28:25–30, 1989

Himle JA, Crystal D, Curtis GC, et al: Mode of onset of simple phobia subtypes: further evidence of heterogeneity. Psychiatry Res 36:37–43, 1991

Hitchcock J, Davis M: Lesions of the amygdala, but not of the cerebellum or red nucleus, block conditioned fear as measured with the potentiated startle paradigm. Behav Neurosis 100:11–22, 1986

Hwu H, Yeh EK, Chang LY: Prevalence of psychiatric disorders in Taiwan defined by the Chinese Diagnostic Interview Schedule. Acta Psychiatr Scand 79:136–147, 1989

Jacobs WJ, Nadel L: Stress-induced recovery of fears and phobias. Psychol Rev 92:512–531, 1985

Kendler KS, Neale MC, Kessler RC, et al: The genetic epidemiology of phobias in women. The interrelationship of agoraphobia, social phobia, situational phobia, and simple phobia. Arch Gen Psychiatry 49:273–281, 1992

Kendler KS, Myers J, Prescott CA: The etiology of phobias: an evaluation of the stress-diathesis model. Arch Gen Psychiatry 59:242–248, 2002

Kessler RC, McGonagle KA, Zhao S, et al: Lifetime and 12-month prevalence of DSM-III-R psychiatric disorders in the United States: results from the National Comorbidity Survey. Arch Gen Psychiatry 51:8–19, 1994

Konorski J: Integrative Activity of the Brain: An Interdisciplinary Approach. Chicago, IL, University of Chicago Press, 1967

Lang PJ: The cognitive psychophysiology of emotion: fear and anxiety, in Anxiety and the Anxiety Disorders. Edited by Tuma AH, Maser JD. Hillsdale, NJ, Lawrence Erlbaum, 1985, pp 131–170

Lang PJ, Davis M, Ohman A: Fear and anxiety: animal models and human cognitive psychophysiology. J Affect Disord 61:137–159, 2000

Lee CK, Kwak YS, Yamamoto J, et al: Psychiatric epidemiology in Korea, I: gender and age differences in Seoul. J Nerv Ment Dis 178:242–246, 1990

Levenson RW: Autonomic nervous system differences among emotions. Psychol Sci 3:23–27, 1992

Liang KC, Melia KR, Campeau S, et al: Lesions of the central nucleus of the amygdala, but not the paraventricular nucleus of the hypothalamus, block the excitatory effects of corticotropin-releasing factor on the acoustic startle reflex. J Neurosci 12:2313–2320, 1992

Magee WJ, Eaton WW, Wittchen HU, et al: Agoraphobia, simple phobia, and social phobia in the National Comorbidity Survey. Arch Gen Psychiatry 53:159–168, 1996

Marks IM: Fear, Phobias, and Rituals: Panic, Anxiety, and Their Disorders. New York, Oxford University Press, 1987

Marshall WL: Behavioral indices of habituation and sensitization during exposure to phobic stimuli. Behav Res Ther 23:167–175, 1988

Matchett G, Davey GC: A test of a disease-avoidance model of animal phobias. Behav Res Ther 29:91–94, 1991

Mathew RJ, Wilson WH, Blazer DG, et al: Psychiatric disorders in adult children of alcoholics: data from the Epidemiologic Catchment Area project. Am J Psychiatry 150:793–800, 1993

Mathews A: Fear-reduction research and clinical phobias. Psychol Bull 85:390–404, 1987

McGaugh JL, Introini-Collison IB, Cahill LF, et al: Neuromodulatory systems and memory storage: role of the amygdala. Behav Brain Res 58:81–90, 1993

Menzies RG, Clarke JC: The etiology of acrophobia and its relationship to severity and individual response patterns. Behav Res Ther 33:795–803, 1995

Muris P, Merckelbach H: How serious are common childhood fears? II: the parent's point of view. Behav Res Ther 38:813–818, 2000

Muris P, Merckelbach H, Schmidt H, et al: Disgust sensitivity, trait anxiety and anxiety disorders symptoms in normal children. Behav Res Ther 37:953–961, 1999a

Muris P, Schmidt H, Merckelbach H: The structure of specific phobia symptoms among children and adolescents. Behav Res Ther 37:863–868, 1999b

Nestadt G, Romanoski AJ, Samuels JF, et al: The relationship between personality and DSM-III Axis I disorders in the population: results from an epidemiological survey. Am J Psychiatry 149:1228–1233, 1992

Okasha A, Omar AM, Lotaief F, et al: Comorbidity of Axis I and Axis II diagnoses in a sample of Egyptian patients with neurotic disorders. Compr Psychiatry 37:95–101, 1996

Ost LG: Blood and injection phobia: background and cognitive, physiological, and behavioral variables. J Abnorm Psychol 101:68–74, 1992

Ost LG, Brandberg M, Alm T: One versus five sessions of exposure in the treatment of flying phobia. Behav Res Ther 35:987–996, 1997

Penick EC, Powell BJ, Nickel EJ, et al: Co-morbidity of lifetime psychiatric disorder among male alcoholic patients. Alcohol Clin Exp Res 18:1289–1293, 1994

Phillips ML, Senior C, Fahy T, et al: Disgust: the forgotten emotion of psychiatry. Br J Psychiatry 172:373–375, 1998

Rachman S, Levitt K, Lopatka C: A simple method for distinguishing between expected and unexpected panics. Behav Res Ther 25:149–154, 1987

Rozin P, Fallon AE: A perspective on disgust. Psychol Rev 94:23–41, 1987

Rudd MD, Dahm PF, Rajab MH: Diagnostic comorbidity in persons with suicidal ideation and behavior. Am J Psychiatry 150:928–934, 1993

Sakanaka M, Shibasaki T, Lederis K: Distribution and efferent projections of corticotropin-releasing factor-like immunoreactivity in the rat amygdaloid complex. Brain Res 382:213–238, 1986

Sanderson WC, Wetzler S, Beck AT, et al: Prevalence of personality disorders among patients with anxiety disorders. Psychiatry Res 51:167–174, 1994

Sareen J, Chartier M, Kjernisted KD, et al: Comorbidity of phobic disorders with alcoholism in a Canadian community sample. Can J Psychiatry 46:733–740, 2001

Seligman ME: Phobias and preparedness. Behav Res Ther 2:307–320, 1971

Shafran R, Booth R, Rachman SJ: The reduction of claustrophobia, II: cognitive analyses. Behav Res Ther 31:75–86, 1993

Starcevic V, Bogojevic G: Comorbidity of panic disorder with agoraphobia and specific phobia: relationship with the subtypes of specific phobia. Compr Psychiatry 38:315–320, 1997

Thyer BA, Himle J, Curtis GC: Blood-injury-illness phobia: a review. J Clin Psychol 41:451–459, 1985

Tillier P, Leclet H, Malgouyres A, et al: [Psychological behavior of patients in MRI: analysis, proposals for improvement and contribution of open magnet equipment] (French). J Radiol 78:433–437, 1997

Tolin DF, Lohr JM, Sawchuk CN, et al: Disgust and disgust sensitivity in blood-injection-injury and spider phobia. Behav Res Ther 35:949–953, 1997

Turner SM, Beidel DC, Borden JW, et al: Social phobia: Axis I and II correlates. J Abnorm Psychol 100:102–106, 1991

van den Hout M, Tenney N, Huygens K, et al: Preconscious processing bias in specific phobia. Behav Res Ther 35:29–34, 1997

Verburg C, Griez E, Meijer J: A 35% carbon dioxide challenge in simple phobias. Acta Psychiatr Scand 90:420–423, 1994

Wik G, Fredrikson M, Fischer H: Cerebral correlates of anticipated fear: a PET study of specific phobia. Int J Neurosci 87:267–276, 1996

World Health Organization: International Statistical Classification of Diseases and Related Health Problems, 10th Revision. Geneva, World Health Organization, 1992

Ziedonis DM, Rayford BS, Bryant KJ, et al: Psychiatric comorbidity in white and African-American cocaine addicts seeking substance abuse treatment. Hosp Community Psychiatry 45:43–49, 1994

Zitrin CM, Klein DF, Woerner MG, et al: Treatment of phobias, I: comparison of imipramine hydrochloride and placebo. Arch Gen Psychiatry 40:125–138, 1983

4

Social Phobia

Franklin R. Schneier, M.D.

Jane A. Luterek, M.A.

Richard G. Heimberg, Ph.D.

Eduardo Leonardo, M.D., Ph.D.

Phenomenology

Symptoms

Social phobia (SP, also known as social anxiety disorder) made its formal appearance in the nomenclature with DSM-III (American Psychiatric Association 1980). Although the original definition emphasized performance-related anxiety, DSM-III-R (American Psychiatric Association 1987) expanded the scope of SP to include individuals whose social fears extended into most social situations. DSM-IV-TR (American Psychiatric Association 2000) defines SP as a marked and persistent fear of one or more social or performance situations in which the person is exposed to unfamiliar people or to scrutiny by others (Table 4–1). The person fears that he or she will behave in a manner that is humiliating or embarrassing and experiences anxiety, which may take the form of a panic attack. The person realizes that the fear is excessive or unreasonable. The fear results in avoidance of situations or severe anxiety in the feared situations, causing functional impairment or marked distress. The symptoms cannot be attributable to a medical disorder or to substance abuse.

Table 4–1.   DSM-IV-TR diagnostic criteria for social phobia

A. A marked and persistent fear of one or more social or performance situations in which the person is exposed to unfamiliar people or to possible scrutiny by others. The individual fears that he or she will act in a way (or show anxiety symptoms) that will be humiliating or embarrassing.   **Note:** In children, there must be evidence of the capacity for age-appropriate social relationships with familiar people and the anxiety must occur in peer settings, not just in interactions with adults.

B. Exposure to the feared social situation almost invariably provokes anxiety, which may take the form of a situationally bound or situationally predisposed panic attack.   **Note:** In children, the anxiety may be expressed by crying, tantrums, freezing, or shrinking from social situations with unfamiliar people.

C. The person recognizes that the fear is excessive or unreasonable.   **Note:** In children, this feature may be absent.

D. The feared social or performance situations are avoided or else are endured with intense anxiety or distress.

E. The avoidance, anxious anticipation, or distress in the feared social or performance situation(s) interferes significantly with the person's normal routine, occupational (academic) functioning, or social activities or relationships, or there is marked distress about having the phobia.

F. In individuals under age 18 years, the duration is at least 6 months.

G. The fear or avoidance is not due to the direct physiological effects of a substance (e.g., a drug of abuse, a medication) or a general medical condition and is not better accounted for by another mental disorder (e.g., panic disorder with or without agoraphobia, separation anxiety disorder, body dysmorphic disorder, a pervasive developmental disorder, or schizoid personality disorder).

H. If a general medical condition or another mental disorder is present, the fear in Criterion A is unrelated to it, e.g., the fear is not of stuttering, trembling in Parkinson's disease, or exhibiting abnormal eating behavior in anorexia nervosa or bulimia nervosa.

Specify if:

   Generalized: if the fears include most social situations (also consider the additional diagnosis of avoidant personality disorder)

DSM-IV-TR subtypes SP along a quantitative spectrum, with the term *generalized* applying to patients who fear most social situations. Individuals with the generalized subtype typically fear and avoid a broad range of both interpersonal and performance situations and often consider themselves to be very shy. Commonly feared interpersonal situations include social gatherings, informal interpersonal contacts (e.g., making small talk with co-workers), behaving assertively, or dealing with authority figures. The generalized subtype is usually more severe, impairing, and associated with more comorbidity, including avoidant personality disorder. The most common form of nongeneralized SP (or "performance anxiety") focuses on fear and avoidance of public speaking. Other situations in which people with SP sometimes fear scrutiny include eating or drinking in public or using public restrooms. There has been some debate over the merits of viewing SP as occurring along a spectrum versus containing separate subtypes.

Those with SP often experience marked anticipatory anxiety prior to feared situations. In social situations, physical symptoms such as palpitations, sweating, blushing, and trembling are common and may become a focus of self-conscious fears of negative evaluation by others. Some people with SP report primarily negative cognitions, with few symptoms of autonomic arousal.

Associated Features

The idea that SP may develop out of a preexisting temperament is supported by studies of children with trait behavioral inhibition. Schwartz et al. (1999) prospectively reevaluated children who had showed arousal and avoidance in response to unfamiliar people or situations in a laboratory evaluation prior to age 3 years, finding increased rates of social anxiety on reevaluation 11 years later. Although onset of SP is often insidious, some patients recall discrete or chronic humiliating experiences as precipitants. In adulthood, SP tends to be highly chronic.

Most people with SP have one or more comorbid disorders (Schneier et al. 1992). Conditions most commonly associated with SP are depression, panic disorder, agoraphobia, generalized anxiety, and substance abuse disorders. In most cases, the diagnosis of SP precedes that of the other diagnosis (Kessler et al. 1999), and the existence of comorbid conditions is associated with a poorer prognosis (Davidson et al. 1993a).

SP is also associated with significant subjective and objective impairment of quality of life. Studies have reported increased suicidal thoughts, poor social supports, poor performance in work and school, and increased use of the health care system (Davidson et al. 1993a; Schneier et al. 1992). People with SP often are limited in school and work achievement by difficulty participating in class or group meetings, being assertive, and dealing with authority figures. They frequently have difficulty initiating friendships and romantic relationships, resulting in limited social relationships and loneliness.

Epidemiology

SP is one of the most common anxiety disorders and is among the most common psychiatric disorders in the general population. Epidemiological and community studies in the United States have estimated the lifetime prevalence to be 2.4%–13.3% (Kessler et al. 1994; Schneier et al. 1992). Older studies that used the narrower DSM-III criteria and probed for fewer social fears tended to produce estimates at the low end of this range. The National Comorbidity Survey estimated 1-year prevalence rates of 7.9% (Kessler et al. 1994) for SP, more than one-half of which appears to represent the generalized subtype.

Epidemiological surveys reveal a higher prevalence in women (Schneier et al. 1992). In clinical samples, however, men and women are more evenly represented. Additionally, people affected with SP are more likely to be single and less educated and to earn less income than their nonaffected peers (Schneier et al. 1992). The age at onset of SP is most commonly in the mid-teens, and in a large majority of cases, the onset of SP occurs by the early 20s (Öst 1987). Many patients, however, report that either their full SP syndrome or subsyndromal shyness was present since early childhood.

Assessment

Differential Diagnosis

When initially evaluating a patient for SP, it is useful to ask general questions about social-evaluative fears, such as "Do you often feel nervous or uncomfortable around others?" and "Do you worry about humiliating or embarrassing yourself in front of others?" Such questions often facilitate discussion of social anxiety symptoms, and the clinician should delineate the specific social situations in which these symptoms occur. The clinician should also attempt to identify the negative thoughts that patients have about the likely outcomes of these situations, their physiological responses of anxiety that occur in these situations, and both active and passive avoidance strategies that may be used to control them. It is important for the clinician to actively probe a wide range of social situations, as patients may be hesitant to report their social anxieties for fear of embarrassment or humiliation in the interview. It is also important to regard patients' reports of inadequate social performance with caution, as it is characteristic of SP to be harshly critical of one's own performance. Self-report, clinician-administered, and behavioral measures may complement the interview to ensure a thorough assessment of SP.

Because empirical treatments specific to SP have been developed, accurate diagnosis is increasingly important. It is sometimes unclear, for example, whether individuals who experience panic attacks and social anxiety or avoidance are best described as having SP or panic disorder (Heimberg and Becker 2002). The primary concern of patients with SP is fear of humiliation or embarrassment, whereas individuals with panic disorder are usually most concerned about the physical and mortal consequences of unexpected panic attacks, and fears of embarrassment or humiliation are secondary. The panic attacks of people with SP are not uncued (or unexpected) and result from fears of being scrutinized or embarrassed by others in specific situations (Jack et al. 1999). Individuals with SP may move away from others for anxiety relief, whereas those with panic disorder may move toward others.

The social withdrawal typical of depression can be similar to the avoidance behavior typical of SP. However, the avoidance behavior of patients with SP is motivated by fears of being scrutinized and negatively evaluated by others; it is an active attempt to avoid an aversive stimulus. In contrast, the social withdrawal of the depressed individual is typically secondary to a lack of energy, lethargy, or anhedonia and is more passive in character.

Assessment Measures

Tools for the assessment of SP have become increasingly sophisticated. This brief review focuses on prominent self-report and clinician-administered measures that have sound psychometric properties and are sensitive to symptom severity and treatment response. We also comment on the utility of cognitive and behavioral assessment in the clinical setting. These measures can be very useful for clinicians in assessing the nature of the patients' presenting symptoms, the severity of the disorder, and the effectiveness of treatment (Hart et al. 1999; McNeil et al. 1995).

Social Interaction Anxiety Scale and Social Phobia Scale

The Social Interaction Anxiety Scale (SIAS) and the Social Phobia Scale (SPS) are commonly used companion self-report measures designed to assess the two different domains of social anxiety: anxiety concerning interpersonal interactions (e.g., initiating and maintaining conversations) and fears of being scrutinized by others in performance situations (e.g., public speaking, eating or drinking in public), respectively (Mattick et al. 1998). Each contains 20 items rated on a scale of 0 ("not at all characteristic or true of me") to 4 ("extremely characteristic or true of me"). Total scores range from 0 to 80; higher scores indicate greater social anxiety. Cutoff scores of 34 for the SIAS and 24 for the SPS differentiate individuals with SP from those without SP (Heimberg et al. 1992). A score of 42 on the SIAS has also been shown to distinguish between people with generalized and those with nongeneralized SP (Mennin et al. 1998). These scales have also been shown to separate patients with SP from those with other anxiety disorders and have been sensitive to the effects of both psychosocial and pharmacological treatments (Brown et al. 1997; Heimberg et al. 1998; Ries et al. 1998).

Social Phobia and Anxiety Inventory

The Social Phobia and Anxiety Inventory (SPAI; Turner et al. 1989) measures specific cognitions, somatic symptoms, avoidance, and escape behavior associated with SP (SP subscale) and anxiety symptoms associated with agoraphobia (agoraphobia subscale). A difference score is calculated by subtracting the agoraphobia score from the SP score. The SPAI contains 45 items, of which 21 items require multiple responses. A total of 109 responses are required of the patient, making the administration of the SPAI more effortful than that of other self-report measures. A cutoff score of 80 on the difference score has been recommended to distinguish SP from other anxiety disorders, and a cutoff score of 60 has been suggested for identifying possible SP for further assessment (Turner et al. 1989). Although the SPAI is a time-consuming measure, it provides a great deal of detail about the nature of the person's SP and may be particularly helpful when the goal is to differentiate between symptoms of SP and those of agoraphobia.

Social Phobia Inventory and Mini-SPIN

The Social Phobia Inventory (SPIN; Connor et al. 2000) assesses fear, avoidance, and physiological symptoms associated with SP. Its 17 items are rated on a 5-point Likert-type scale ranging from 0 ("not at all") to 4 ("extremely"), with a total score ranging from 0 to 68. A cutoff score of 19 was found to distinguish between individuals with SP and those without it (Connor et al. 2000). This measure assesses physiological symptoms associated with SP (an area that is not well sampled by the other scales). Connor et al. (2001) also evaluated the utility of the Mini-SPIN, which consists of three items from the original SPIN. The Mini-SPIN has been a very effective tool for identifying individuals with and without generalized SP in a managed care setting and may be useful in other psychiatric and psychological settings, though further research is needed.

Clinician-Rated Instruments

The Liebowitz Social Anxiety Scale (LSAS; Liebowitz 1987) and Brief Social Phobia Scale (Davidson et al. 1997) are clinician-administered scales for the assessment of SP. Here we review the more frequently employed LSAS. The LSAS separately evaluates fear and avoidance of 11 social (e.g., talking to people in authority) and 13 performance (e.g., telephoning in public) situations on a 4-point Likert-type scale. Recent empirical work also suggests that the LSAS can be administered as a self-report measure without compromising the reliability and validity of the measure when clear instructions are provided (Fresco et al. 2001). The LSAS contains four subscales (social fear, performance fear, social avoidance, and performance avoidance) and three total scores with a total fear score, a total avoidance score, and an overall total score. Recent empirical research suggests that a cutoff score of 30 on the LSAS total score differentiates individuals with SP from those without it and that a total score of 60 distinguishes individuals with generalized SP from those without it (Mennin et al. 2002). Although the LSAS provides a thorough assessment of SP fear and avoidance symptoms across various situations and can be a useful diagnostic tool, it can be particularly valuable in identifying social and performance situations that should be the target of treatment.

Assessment of Cognition in Social Phobia

Assessment of SP should routinely include attention to the thoughts that patients report in social situations. These may be assessed via interview, but it is often useful to supplement the interview with questionnaires such as the Brief

Fear of Negative Evaluation Scale (Leary 1983) or the Social Interaction Self-Statement Test (Glass et al. 1982). Heimberg and Becker (2002) and Hart et al. (1999) have provided more detailed information on these measures and other approaches to cognitive assessment of SP.

Behavioral Assessment Tests

An important part of the assessment of patients with SP is an evaluation of the adequacy of their social behavior. Individuals with SP judge their own performance more harshly than others (Rapee and Lim 1992) and overestimate the visibility of their anxiety (Alden and Wallace 1995), so self-reports of the quality of their social behavior are unlikely to be veridical. Neither is observation of behavior in the protected interview setting likely to provide detail about the quality of social performance or the visibility of anxiety symptoms in feared social settings. Behavioral assessment tests (BATs) can provide that information.

BATs are brief role-plays in which the patient encounters a mock-up of a fear-eliciting social situation. Common BATs include giving a speech to a small audience and conversations with same- or opposite-gender strangers. However, to be most clinically useful, the BAT should be tailored to the needs of the individual patient, incorporating specific stimuli that the patient fears. For instance, if a patient fears confrontations with authority figures, the BAT could involve asking the patient to role-play speaking with his or her boss, with the goal being to ask for a raise in pay.

Role-plays can be conducted between therapist and patient or by using other personnel if available. The patient's anxiety can easily be assessed by asking for 0–100 ratings at regular intervals, and the presence/absence or quality of component social behaviors (e.g., eye contact, posture, voice volume, verbal content) can be examined as well. Although BATs may not be commonly used in clinical practice, they can provide invaluable information that may not be available from other types of assessments.

Pathogenesis

Biological

Family and twin studies suggest significant genetic and environmental contributions to the development of SP. First-degree relatives of patients with SP have increased rates of SP (Fyer et al. 1993), but this familiality may be limited to patients with the generalized subtype (Stein et al. 1998a). Kendler et al. (1992) reported, on the basis of data from 2,163 directly interviewed female twins, that 30%–40% of SP is heritable. A follow-up study, reinterviewing 1,708 of the original cohort, resulted in an estimate of a 51% genetic contribution (Kendler et al. 1999). A smaller study showed no increase in rates of SP between monozygotic twins (Skre et al. 1993).

Patients with SP experience signs of autonomic arousal when in social settings. This observation led to the hypothesis that patients with SP may have an overactive autonomic nervous system. Levin et al. (1993) examined the heart rate and blood pressure response to a public speaking task of patients with SP and control subjects. Surprisingly, patients with generalized SP did not differ from control subjects in these physiological parameters. Further studies have confirmed these findings (Naftolowitz et al. 1994) and have suggested that only SP limited to performance anxiety may be associated with increased autonomic reactivity.

Dopaminergic transmission has been postulated to play a role in SP. Patients with SP appear to show a preferential response to monoamine oxidase inhibitors (MAOIs), which have dopaminergic activity, and lower levels of dopamine metabolites in the cerebrospinal fluid have been associated with introversion. Recent functional brain imaging studies have found decreased striatal dopamine D_2 receptor and dopamine transporter binding in patients with SP (Schneier and Altieri 2003). Dopamine circuits mediating social reward have been postulated to be dysfunctional in SP.

Differences have been shown in several other brain systems in patients with SP. Neurohormonal studies have found some evidence for serotonin and growth hormone abnormalities. Functional magnetic resonance imaging studies of amygdala function have suggested that a sensitivity to fear conditioning may be present in SP (Argyropoulos et al. 2001).

Psychosocial

Because SP involves fears of negative evaluation and embarrassment in social situations, it is not surprising that psychosocial aspects of childhood and adolescence play a significant role in the pathogenesis of this disorder. Empirical research has suggested that modeling, restricted exposure to social situations, the nature of the family environment, and peer relations may be influential in the development of SP (Roth et al., in press).

Individuals learn how to relate to their social environment largely through their parents or caretakers. Thus, the fears experienced by individuals with SP may arise, in part, from modeling their parents' social behavior. Individuals with SP often grow up with parents who have strong social-evaluative concerns, placing great importance on making a good impression with others (Bruch et al. 1989; Caster et al. 1999). This emphasis may encourage children to overestimate the standards expected by others or the negative consequences of not meeting these standards, leading to increased expectation of threat in social situations (Bruch et al. 1989; Buss 1980; Cloitre and Shear 1995). Parents may also model their own social anxiety to their children, further communicating to them that the social world is a dangerous place and promoting the belief that the social environment should be feared. This may lead children to be more likely to notice social threat in their environment and promote the avoidance of social situations.

Parental social behaviors that restrict children's exposure to rewarding social relations may also encourage the development of SP. Parents who are restricted in their own social relations and/or do not foster social activities in which their children may interact with others facilitate social avoidance and prevent the extinction of naturally occurring social fears in their children (Bruch et al. 1989). As a result, the children may have less opportunity to develop the interpersonal skills necessary for rewarding social relationships and may be more likely than other children to view interactions with peers as punishing rather than pleasurable.

In addition, childhood exposure to parenting styles that are overprotective (e.g., Lieb et al. 2000), involve little display of affection toward the child (e.g., Arrindell et al. 1989), and use shame as a method of discipline (Bruch and Heimberg 1994) is frequently reported among adolescents and adults with SP. Excessive parental control may inadvertently convey to children that they are inept, whereas decreased levels of parental affection and the use of shame may increase perceptions that other people are critical and that negative evaluation is a likely outcome of social situations.

This perception also may have been developed and/or reinforced through peer relations, especially as children grow older and spend more time with peers than family members. Interpersonal experiences with peers may serve to exacerbate and maintain symptoms of social anxiety; however, this relationship seems to be reciprocal. On the one hand, passive and withdrawn children are more likely to be rejected by their peers, which may contribute to the development of a belief that they cannot succeed in the social world, resulting in increased social avoidance behavior (Rubin and Mills 1988). On the other hand, socially anxious children are more likely than nonanxious children to experience negative peer relations, and these experiences, most notably peer neglect (La Greca et al. 1988; Strauss et al. 1988), may contribute to the maintenance of social anxiety. Adults with SP also report having been teased and bullied during childhood, suggesting that these difficulties with peers can continue to have an impact into adulthood (McCabe et al. 2000; Roth et al. 2002).

Although we have focused here on family environment and peer relations in the development and maintenance of SP, the underlying theme is the perception that the social world is a harsh and critical place. The prominent fear of negative evaluation in SP may have arisen from parenting practices or social experiences that directly or indirectly promote this belief, coupled with the facilitation of social avoidance strategies that reduce the likelihood of rewarding relationships that could alter this perception. In fact, socially anxious people demonstrate a number of beliefs of this nature, including the belief that others are highly critical (Leary et al. 1988), that others hold high but often unarticulated standards for their performance (Alden and Wallace 1991), and that social success leads only to higher expectations for performance in the future (Wallace and Alden 1997).

Pharmacotherapy

Selective Serotonin Reuptake Inhibitors

Selective serotonin reuptake inhibitors (SSRIs) have emerged as a first-line pharmacotherapy for SP, on the basis of efficacy in several large placebo-controlled trials. Response rates, with response generally defined by scores of 1 or 2 ("much or very much improved") on the Clinical Global Impression Improvement Scale, have ranged from 40% to 70% for active drug versus 8%–32% for placebo. For example, Stein et al. (1998b) reported on 187 patients with SP treated with paroxetine (mean dose, 37 mg/day) or placebo for 12 weeks in a double-blind study. They reported a 55% response rate to paroxetine, compared with a 24% rate for placebo. Van Ameringen et al. (2001) randomly assigned 204 patients with SP to receive sertraline or placebo, obtaining a 53% response rate to sertraline (mean dose, 146 mg/day) versus 29% response to placebo at the end of 20 weeks. A randomized trial also exists for fluvoxamine (43% response rate vs. 23% placebo response; Stein et al. 1999). Open trials of citalopram suggest efficacy in SP similar to the other SSRIs (e.g., Bouwer and Stein 1998), but open trials suggesting efficacy for fluoxetine were not support by a recent controlled trial (Kobak et al. 2002).

The doses of SSRIs used in these studies are similar to those used in the treatment of depression. As with the treatment of depression, there appears to be a lag between initiation of medication and treatment response. Treatment with medication appears to separate from placebo at about 6–8 weeks, with continued improvement on medication for up to 20 weeks (Van Ameringen et al. 2001). SSRI trials, like most clinical trials for SP, have included a preponderance of patients with the generalized subtype, so it remains unclear to what extent the results apply to patients with nongeneralized SP.

Benzodiazepines

Benzodiazepines have long been used clinically for SP, although controlled trials have been conducted only for clonazaepam and alprazolam given on a daily basis. Several open-label studies (e.g., Munjack et al. 1990) and a double-blind placebo-controlled trial (Davidson et al. 1993b) support the efficacy of clonazepam for SP. The controlled trial found a 78% response rate after 10 weeks of clonazepam versus a 20% response rate on placebo. Mean clonazepam dose at the end of the study was 2.4 mg/day, with a range of 0.5 mg–3.0 mg. Otto et al. (2000) conducted a 12-week study comparing clonazepam to group cognitive-behavioral therapy (CBT). The results suggested that both patient populations improved similarly, with clonazepam showing better efficacy on some measures at 12 weeks. The data for alprazolam include a couple of promising open-label studies (e.g., Lydiard et al. 1988) and one negative double-blind placebo-controlled study (Gelernter et al. 1991).

Limitations of treatment with benzodiazepines in SP include their contraindication in the presence of comorbid substance abuse, lack of specific efficacy for comorbid depression, and potential for dependency. Clonazepam, however, does not appear to be difficult for patients with SP to discontinue. Connor et al. (1998) randomly assigned responders after 6 months of clonazepam treatment to continued treatment or a discontinuation taper by 0.25 mg every 2 weeks. Relapse rates were 0% in the continuation group and 21%

in the discontinuation group after 5 months of follow-up monitoring. The finding that most patients in the discontinuation group maintained their response suggests that short-term (6-month) treatment followed by slow taper may be a reasonable treatment option.

The alternative dosing of benzodiazepines on an as-needed basis, although not formally studied in SP, may have utility in the nongeneralized subtype when feared situations are occasional and predictable. Some patients may experience sedation and/or cognitive impairment at anxiolytic as-needed dosages, however, so β-adrenergic blockers have tended to be favored clinically for as-needed dosing of anxiety in predictable performance situations.

Monoamine Oxidase Inhibitors

MAOIs have well-established efficacy for SP but have become second-line agents because of the risk of hypertensive reactions and the inconvenience of dietary restrictions.

Four double-blind placebo-controlled trials describe the effectiveness of phenelzine in SP. For example, Liebowitz et al. (1992) randomly assigned 85 patients with SP to receive phenelzine, atenolol, or placebo for 8 weeks. Among patients who completed at least 4 weeks of treatment, 64% responded to phenelzine (mean dose, 75.7 mg/day) compared with a 30% response to atenolol and a 23% response to placebo. (See also Gelernter et al. 1991; Heimberg et al. 1998; Versiani et al. 1992.) Open-trial data suggest that other MAOIs, particularly tranylcypromine, may also have efficacy for SP.

Reversible MAOIs have attracted interest as possible therapeutic agents for SP because of their decreased risk of causing a hypertensive reaction. Controlled trials have suggested that brofaromine is effective, but results for moclobemide are mixed, and neither is marketed in the United States at this time.

β-Adrenergic Blockers

Anecdotal evidence as well as controlled trials in nonclinical samples suggest that β-blockers used on an as-needed basis may be helpful in situations related to specific performance anxiety. β-blockers may be particularly useful for people with prominent symptoms of autonomic arousal, including palpitations and hand tremor. Clinically, it appears that a dose of 10–40 mg of propranolol taken about 1 hour before a performance is sufficient for many patients. The drug is generally well tolerated by healthy adults, but trying a test dose prior to the performance day can be reassuring to the patient. Controlled trials of daily dosing with β-blockers in predominantly generalized SP samples have not supported their usefulness for generalized SP. β-blockers are contraindicated in patients with asthma and some cardiac conditions.

Buspirone

Data supporting the use of buspirone in the treatment of SP have been mixed. Two randomized placebo-controlled trials showed no benefit over placebo (Clark and Agras 1991; van Vliet et al. 1997). However, both of these studies used fixed daily doses of 30 mg that were below doses used in several open-label trials that suggested efficacy (e.g., Schneier et al. 1993). Buspirone also may be a useful adjunct to treatment with SSRIs.

Other Medications

The use of gabapentin in patients with generalized SP is supported by one placebo-controlled 14-week study (Pande et al. 1999). The study demonstrated a statistically significant decrease in social anxiety (LSAS) scores in gabapentin-treated subjects compared with control subjects, but no statistically significant difference in response rates. Most responders took doses toward the upper end of the range of 900–3,600 mg/day.

Several antidepressant medications have been studied for SP in only open trials. Open-label studies suggest that venlafaxine may be effective in treating symptoms of SP (e.g., Altamura et al. 1999). An open-label study of bupropion treatment of 18 patients (Emmanuel et al. 2000) reported that 50% of patients completing the study were responders. Van Ameringen et al. (1999) reported a 70% response rate to nefazodone in a 12-week open trial. Tricyclic antidepressants, however, have appeared ineffective in the treatment of SP (Simpson et al. 1998).

Because pharmacotherapy response in SP is often partial, augmentation is frequently considered. Few data are available. Buspirone has been suggested to have efficacy in augmenting SSRIs, and clonazepam is commonly used for this purpose as well. MAOIs, however, should not be used in conjunction with SSRIs or buspirone. CBT and other psychotherapies are commonly combined with medications in an attempt to augment benefits and protect against relapse when medication is discontinued.

Psychotherapy

Cognitive-behavioral therapy is the most extensively researched and empirically supported of the several different psychotherapies that have been applied to the treatment of SP, including interpersonal (Lipsitz et al. 1999), psychodynamic (Gabbard 1992), and Morita therapies (Reynolds 1980). CBT is a time-limited, present-oriented approach to psychotherapy aimed at increasing the patient's range of cognitive and behavioral skills in a collaborative working relationship between patient and therapist. A large number of techniques fall under the rubric of CBT. However, a limited number have proven beneficial for the amelioration of social anxiety. These are reviewed in the following sections.

Exposure

Exposure is designed to assist the patient in confronting feared situations while staying psychologically engaged, allowing the natural conditioning processes involved in fear reduction (habituation and extinction) to occur. The patient, in collaboration with the therapist, begins the process of exposure by constructing a *fear hierarchy*, a rank-ordered list of anxiety-provoking social situations. The fear hierarchy typically includes the patient's ratings of the amount of anxiety that he or she would experience in the situation and the degree to which he or she avoids the situations in everyday life. Once the fear hierarchy is constructed, the patient starts with the least-feared social situation and progressively moves up the list to more-feared situations as less-feared situations are mastered. Exposures are conducted using the following three different methods, typically in combination: imaginal (as the therapist narrates scenes for the patient to imagine), role-play (during the therapy session), and confrontation of feared situations (outside of session).

For exposures to be maximally effective, it is essential that the patient pay full attention to the details of the anxiety-provoking situation, to experience it fully and allow the inevitable rush of anxiety and arousal to occur (Foa and Kozak 1986). However, patients often attempt to divert their attention or think about other things in an effort to manage their anxiety, which inadvertently undermines the potential effectiveness of the exposure. Instructing patients to pay full attention to the situation during exposure exercises facilitates the effectiveness of this therapeutic technique (Wells and Papageorgiou 1998).

Cognitive Restructuring

Recent cognitive-behavioral models (Clark and Wells 1995; Rapee and Heimberg 1997) suggest that cognitive factors are central to the development and maintenance of SP. Specifically, patients' fears are proposed to arise from inaccurate beliefs about the potential dangers of social situations, predictions about the negative outcomes of these situations, and biased processing of events that occur during social situations.

Contemporary cognitive-behavioral approaches to therapy for social anxiety are centered on the technique of cognitive restructuring, derived from Beck and Emery's (1985) approach to cognitive therapy and Ellis's (1962) rational emotive therapy. In cognitive restructuring, patients are taught to identify negative thoughts that occur before, during, or after confronting the feared situation. Next, in collaboration with the therapist, patients evaluate the accuracy of these thoughts using evidence obtained through Socratic dialogue and/or as a result of planned exposures. Once the collected data are evaluated, the patient and therapist derive rational alternative thoughts. The use of rational alternative thoughts, instead of their habitual negative interpretations, provides the patient with a cognitive coping strategy for anxiety-provoking situations. Exposures are a key component of cognitive restructuring, as they provide the opportunities for patients to assess whether their negative beliefs are realistic or anxiogenic and to practice using rational alternative responses.

Thus, exposures are used in this context to undermine the negative beliefs that patients have about social situations and to provide evidence in favor of more adaptive alternatives. For instance, a patient may have the belief that "I will not be able to speak" or "no one will be interested in what I have to say" if he or she contributes to a discussion in a meeting at work. The patient may be asked to participate in a work-related discussion (by imagining the unfolding of the event, by role-playing in the therapy session, or by attending and participating in the actual event) and gather evidence to evaluate these beliefs. Another critical element of the use of exposures in cognitive restructuring is to require the patient to enter the anxiety-provoking situation without engaging in his or her habitual "safety behaviors" (Wells et al. 1995). For example, a patient may look down while talking during a meeting at work, or carefully rehearse what he or she will say, as a way to reduce anxiety and also to reduce the likelihood of the feared result (e.g., not being able to speak, other people not being interested). Patients often attribute successful outcomes to their use of safety behaviors (e.g., carefully rehearsing what to say resulted in being able to speak and in others being interested). Therefore, it is important for patients to assess whether the feared consequences actually happen without their engaging in the safety behaviors. Within cognitive restructuring, exposures provide opportunities for the patients to receive corrective information about the accuracy of their beliefs and to practice rational alternatives that are more adaptive than their habitual negative thoughts.

Relaxation Training

Individuals with SP often experience an excessive amount of physiological arousal in anticipation of and during feared situations, and this arousal may interfere with optimal social performance. Relaxation training provides patients with a means of coping with the physiological component of social anxiety. Current relaxation techniques, derived from the pioneering work of Wolpe (1958) and Bernstein and Borkovec (1973; see also Bernstein et al. 2000), involve relaxation exercises focusing on different muscle groups that are practiced in and outside of sessions. The patient is asked to focus on a particular muscle group, tensing it and then releasing the tension for 5–10 seconds while examining the differences in sensation produced from tensing and relaxing. Typically, relaxation training involves first working on 16 different muscle groups and then focusing on larger muscle groups to achieve more rapid relaxation. Relaxation training may also involve cue-controlled relaxation, in which a word (e.g., *relax*, *calm*) is repeatedly paired with a relaxed bodily state. This technique allows the patient to use the word as a cue to achieve feelings of relaxation during everyday activities. These relaxation techniques are most effective for patients with SP if they are ultimately applied during anxiety-provoking social situations. Applied relaxation combines relaxation techniques with exposures to feared situations (Öst 1987). It involves targeting the following three skill areas in treatment: 1) learning to attend to the physiological arousal of anxiety, 2) quickly relaxing while engaging in everyday activities, and 3) applying these relaxation techniques, when a high level of skill has been achieved, in anxiety-provoking situations.

Social Skills Training

Social skills training is predicated on the assumption that individuals with SP lack knowledge of or adequate skills to perform the behaviors necessary for successful social interaction. As a result, they elicit negative reactions from others, and social interactions become both punishing and anxiety-provoking. The obvious implication of this position is that psychological therapy must facilitate effective social performance. However, the reasons for poor social performance are often unclear. It *may* result from deficits in social skill, but inhibition or disruption of behavior by anxiety, maladaptive thoughts, physiological arousal, or a combination of these or other factors provide alternative explanations. In our clinic, it is not uncommon for patients to report that they do not know how to behave, even though observation reveals otherwise. (See the earlier discussion about the importance of behavioral assessment). Nevertheless, social skills training, which typically involves therapist modeling, behavioral rehearsal, corrective feedback, social reinforcement, and homework assignments, may benefit a number of patients. Whether or not it remediates deficits in the patient's social repertoire, it may provide benefits due to the exposure elements (e.g., confrontation of the feared social situation through homework assignments) or the cognitive elements (e.g., corrective feedback about the competence of one's social behavior) inherent in this intervention.

Conclusion

CBT has proved to be an efficacious treatment for SP. Gains achieved in CBT appear to be durable (Heimberg et al. 1993), with some studies showing additional improvements in the months following the discontinuation of treatment (Taylor 1996). Although there have been few studies comparing CBT and pharmacological interventions, the literature to date suggests that CBT may provide better protection from relapse, although medications may offer somewhat greater initial symptom relief (Heimberg 2001). Little is known about the utility of combining pharmacological and CBT approaches, although this strategy is frequently employed. In sum, CBT offers patients a time-limited approach that has proven efficacy in reducing social anxiety symptoms and may be a useful alternative or complement to pharmacological interventions.

References

Agyropoulos SV, Bell CJ, Nutt DJ: Brain function in social anxiety disorder. Psychiatr Clin North Am 24:707–722, 2001

Alden LE, Wallace ST: Social standards and social withdrawal. Cognit Ther Res 15:85–100, 1991

Alden LE, Wallace ST: Social phobia and social appraisal in successful and unsuccessful social interactions. Behav Res Ther 33:497–505, 1995

Altamura AC, Pioli R, Vitto M, et al: Venlafaxine in social phobia: a study in selective serotonin reuptake inhibitor non-responders. Int Clin Psychopharmacol 14:239–45, 1999

American Psychiatric Association: Diagnostic and Statistical Manual of Mental Disorders, 3rd Edition. Washington, DC, American Psychiatric Association, 1980

American Psychiatric Association: Diagnostic and Statistical Manual of Mental Disorders, 3rd Edition, Revised. Washington, DC, American Psychiatric Association, 1987

American Psychiatric Association: Diagnostic and Statistical Manual of Mental Disorders, 4th Edition, Text Revision. Washington, DC, American Psychiatric Association, 2000

Arrindell WA, Kwee MGT, Methorst GJ, et al: Perceived parental rearing styles of agoraphobic and social phobic inpatients. Br J Psychiatry 155:526–535, 1989

Beck AT, Emery G: Anxiety Disorders and Phobias: A Cognitive Perspective. New York, Basic Books, 1985

Bernstein DA, Borkovec TD: Progressive Relaxation Training: A Manual for the Helping Professions. Champaign, IL, Research Press, 1973

Bernstein DA, Borkovec TD, Hazlett-Stevens H: New Directions in Progressive Relaxation Training: A Guidebook for Helping Professionals. Westport, CT, Praeger, 2000

Bouwer C, Stein DJ: Use of the selective serotonin reuptake inhibitor citalopram in the treatment of generalized social phobia. J Affect Disord 49:79–82, 1998

Brown EJ, Turovsky J, Heimberg R, et al: Validation of the Social Interaction Anxiety Scale and the Social Phobia Scale across the anxiety disorders. Psychol Assess 9:21–27, 1997

Bruch MA, Heimberg RG: Differences in perceptions of parental and personal characteristics between generalized and nongeneralized social phobics. J Anxiety Disord 8:155–168, 1994

Bruch MA, Heimberg RG, Berger P, et al: Social phobia and perceptions of early parental and personal characteristics. Anxiety Res 2:57–65, 1989

Buss AH: Self-Consciousness and Social Anxiety. San Francisco, CA, Freeman, 1980

Caster JB, Inderbitzen HM, Hope D: Relationship between youth and parent perceptions of family environment and social anxiety. J Anxiety Disord 13:237–251, 1999

Clark D, Agras WS: The assessment and treatment of performance anxiety in musicians. Am J Psychiatry 148:598–605, 1991

Clark DM, Wells A: A cognitive model of social phobia, in Social Phobia: Diagnosis, Assessment, and Treatment. Edited by Heimberg RG, Liebowitz MR, Hope DA, et al. New York, Guilford, 1995, pp 69–93

Cloitre M, Shear MK: Psychodynamic perspectives, in Social Phobia: Clinical and Research Perspectives. Edited by MB Stein. Washington, DC, American Psychiatric Press, 1995, pp 163–187

Connor KM, Davidson JR, Potts NL, et al: Discontinuation of clonazepam in the treatment of social phobia. J Clin Psychopharmacol 18:373–378, 1998

Connor KM, Davidson JRT, Churchill LE, et al: Psychometric properties of the Social Phobia Inventory (SPIN): a new self-rating scale. Br J Psychiatry 176:379–386, 2000

Connor KM, Kobak KA, Churchill LE, et al: Mini-SPIN: a brief screening assessment for generalized social anxiety disorder. Depress Anxiety 14:137–140, 2001

Davidson JRT, Hughes DL, George LK, et al: The epidemiology of social phobia: findings from the Duke Epidemiological Catchment Area Study. Psychol Med 23:709–718, 1993a

Davidson JRT, Potts NLS, Richichi E, et al: Treatment of social phobia with clonazepam and placebo. J Clin Psychopharmacol 13:423–428, 1993b

Davidson JRT, Miner CM, DeVeaugh-Geiss J, et al: The Brief Social Phobia Scale: a psychometric evaluation. Psychol Med 27:161–166, 1997

Ellis A: Reason and Emotion in Psychotherapy. New York, Lyle Stuart, 1962

Emmanuel NP, Brawman-Mintzer O, Morton WA, et al: Bupropion-SR in treatment of social phobia. Depress Anxiety 12:111–113, 2000

Fresco DM, Coles ME, Heimberg RG, et al: The Liebowitz Social Anxiety Scale: a comparison of the psychometric properties of self-report and clinician-administered formats. Psychol Med 31:1025–1035, 2001

Foa EB, Kozak MJ: Emotional processing of fear: exposure to corrective information. Psychol Bull 99:20–35, 1986

Fyer AJ, Mannuzza S, Chapman TF, et al: A direct interview family study of social phobia. Arch Gen Psychiatry 50:286–293, 1993

Gabbard GO: Psychodynamics of panic disorder and social phobia. Bull Menninger Clin 56:A3–A13, 1992

Gelernter CS, Uhde TW, Cimbolic P, et al: Cognitive-behavioral and pharmacological treatments of social phobia. Arch Gen Psychiatry 48:938–945, 1991

Glass CR, Merluzzi TV, Biever JL, et al: Cognitive assessment of social anxiety: development and validation of a self-statement questionnaire. Cognit Ther Res 6:37–55, 1982

Hart TA, Jack MS, Turk CL, et al: Issues for the measurement of social anxiety disorder (social phobia), in Focus on Psychiatry: Social Anxiety Disorder. Edited by Westenberg HGM, Den Boer JA. Amsterdam, Netherlands, Syn-Thesis Publishers, 1999

Heimberg RG: Current status of psychotherapeutic interventions for social phobia. J Clin Psychiatry 62 (suppl):36–42, 2001

Heimberg RG, Becker RE: Cognitive-Behavioral Treatment for Social Phobia: Basic Mechanisms and Clinical Strategies. New York, Guilford, 2002

Heimberg RG, Mueller GP, Holt CS, et al: Assessment of anxiety in social interaction and being observed by others: the Social Interaction Anxiety Scale and the Social Phobia Scale. Behav Ther 23:53–73, 1992

Heimberg RG, Salzman D, Holt CS, et al: Cognitive behavioral group treatment of social phobia: effectiveness at 5-year follow-up. Cognit Ther Res 17:325–339, 1993

Heimberg RG, Liebowitz MR, Hope DA, et al: Cognitive behavioral group therapy vs. phenelzine therapy for social phobia: 12-week outcome. Arch Gen Psychiatry 55:1133–1141, 1998

Jack MS, Heimberg RG, Mennin DS: Situational panic attacks: impact on social phobia with and without panic disorder. Depress Anxiety 10:112–118, 1999

Kendler KS, Neale MC, Kessler RC, et al: The genetic epidemiology of phobias in women. The interrelationship of agoraphobia, social phobia, situational phobia, and simple phobia. Arch Gen Psychiatry 49:273–281, 1992

Kendler KS, Karkowski LM, Prescott CA: Fears and phobias: reliability and heritability. Psychol Med 29:529–553, 1999

Kessler RC, McGonagle KA, Zhao S, et al: Lifetime and 12-month prevalence of DSM-III-R psychiatric disorders in the United States: results from the National Comorbidity Survey. Arch Gen Psychiatry 51:8–19, 1994

Kessler RC, Stang P, Wittchen H-U, et al: Lifetime co-morbidities between social phobia and mood disorders in the US National Comorbidity Survey. Psychol Med 29:555–567, 1999

Kobak DA, Griest JH, Jefferson JW, et al: Fluoxetine in social phobia: a double-blind, placebo-controlled pilot study. J Clin Psychopharmacol 22:257–262, 2002

La Greca AM, Dandes SK, Wick P, et al: Development of the social anxiety scale for children: reliability and concurrent validity. J Child Clin Psychol 17:84–91, 1988

Leary MR: A brief version of the Fear of Negative Evaluation Scale. Pers Soc Psychol Bull 9:371–375, 1983

Leary MR, Kowalski RM, Campbell CD: Self-presentational concerns and social anxiety: the role of generalized impression expectancies. J Res Pers 22:308–321, 1988

Levin AP, Saoud JB, Strauman T, et al: Responses of "generalized" and "discrete" social phobics during public speaking. J Anxiety Disord 7:207–221, 1993

Lieb R, Wittchen HU, Höfler M, et al: Parental psychopathology, parenting styles, and the risk of social phobia in offspring. Arch Gen Psychiatry 57:859–866, 2000

Liebowitz MR: Social phobia. Mod Probl Pharmacopsychiatry 22:141–173, 1987

Liebowitz MR, Schneier FR, Campeas R, et al: Phenelzine versus atenolol in social phobia: a placebo-controlled comparison. Arch Gen Psychiatry 49:290–300, 1992

Lipsitz JD, Markowitz JC, Cherry S, et al: Open trial of interpersonal psychotherapy for the treatment of social phobia. Am J Psychiatry 156:1814–1816, 1999

Lydiard RB, Laraia MT, Howell EF, et al: Alprazolam in the treatment of social phobia. J Clin Psychiatry 49:17–19, 1988

Mattick RP, Peters L, Clarke JC: Exposure and cognitive restructuring for social phobia: a controlled study. Behav Ther 20:3–23, 1989

McCabe RE, Liss AL, Summerfeldt LJ, et al: An examination of the relation between anxiety disorders and self-reported history of teasing or bullying experience during adolescence and childhood. Paper presented at the annual meeting of the Association for the Advancement of Behavior Therapy, New Orleans, LA, November 2000

McNeil DW, Ries BJ, Turk CL: Behavioral assessment: self-report, physiology, and overt behavior, in Social Phobia: Diagnosis, Assessment, and Treatment. Edited by Heimberg RG, Liebowitz MR, Hope DA, et al. New York, Guilford, 1995, pp 202–231

Mennin DS, Fresco DM, Heimberg RG: Determining subtype of social phobia in a clinical setting: validation using a receiver operating characteristic (ROC) analysis. Paper presented at the annual meeting of the Association for Advancement of Behavior Therapy, Washington, DC, November 1998

Mennin DS, Fresco DM, Heimberg RG, et al: Screening for social anxiety disorder in the clinical setting using the Liebowitz Social Anxiety Scale. J Anxiety Disord 16:661–673, 2002

Munjack DJ, Baltazar PL, Bohn PB, et al: Clonazepam in the treatment of social phobia: a pilot study. J Clin Psychiatry 51 (suppl 5):35–40, 1990

Naftolowitz DF, Vaughn BV, Ranc J, et al: Response to alcohol in social phobia. Anxiety 1:96–99, 1994

Ontiveros A, Fontaine R: Social phobia and clonazepam. Can J Psychiatry 35:439–441, 1990

Öst LG: Applied relaxation: description of a coping technique and review of controlled studies. Behav Res Ther 25:397–409, 1987

Otto MW, Pollack MH, Gould RA, et al: A comparison of the efficacy of clonazepam and cognitive-behavioral group therapy for the treatment of social phobia. J Anxiety Disord 14:345–358, 2000

Pande AC, Davidson JR, Jefferson JW, et al: Treatment of social phobia with gabapentin: a placebo-controlled study. J Clin Psychopharmacol 19:341–348, 1999

Rapee RM, Heimberg RG: A cognitive-behavioral model of anxiety in social phobia. Behav Res Ther 35:741–756, 1997

Rapee RM, Lim L: Discrepancy between self- and observer ratings of performance in social phobics. J Abnorm Psychol 101:728–731, 1992

Reynolds DK: The Quiet Therapies. Honolulu, University of Hawaii Press, 1980

Ries BJ, McNeil DW, Boone ML, et al: Assessment of contemporary social phobia verbal report instruments. Behav Res Ther 36:983–994, 1998

Roth DA, Coles ME, Heimberg RG: The relationship between memories for childhood teasing and anxiety and depression in adulthood. J Anxiety Disord 16:149–164, 2002

Roth DA, Fresco DM, Heimberg RG: Cognitive phenomena in social anxiety disorder, in Cognitive Vulnerability to Emotional Disorders. Edited by Alloy LB, Riskind JH. Hillsdale, NJ, Lawrence Erlbaum (in press)

Rubin KH, Mills RSL: The many faces of social isolation in children. J Consult Clin Psychol 56:916–924, 1988

Schneier FR, Altieri PI: Imaging dopamine system function in personality traits and generalized social phobia, in Dopamine Receptors and Transporters, 2nd Edition. Edited by Sidgu A, Laruelle M, Vernier P. New York, Marcel Dekker, 2003, pp 705–729

Schneier FR, Johnson J, Hornig CD, et al: Social phobia: comorbidity and morbidity in an epidemiologic sample. Arch Gen Psychiatry 49:282–288, 1992

Schneier FR, Saoud JB, Campeas R, et al: Buspirone in social phobia. J Clin Psychopharmacol 13:251–256, 1993

Schwartz CE, Snidman N, Kagan J: Adolescent social anxiety as an outcome of inhibited temperament in childhood. J Am Acad Child Adolesc Psychiatry 38:1008–1016, 1999

Simpson HB, Schneier FR, Campeas RB, et al: Imipramine in the treatment of social phobia. J Clin Psychopharmacol 18:132–135, 1998

Skre I, Onstad S, Torgersen S, et al: A twin study of DSM-III-R anxiety disorders. Acta Psychiatr Scand 88:85–92, 1993

Stein MB, Chartier MJ, Hazen AL, et al: A direct-interview family study of generalized social phobia. Am J Psychiatry 155:90–97, 1998a

Stein MB, Liebowitz MR, Lydiard B, et al: Paroxetine treatment of generalized social phobia (social anxiety disorder): a randomized controlled trial. JAMA 280:708–713, 1998b

Stein MB, Fyer AJ, Davidson JRT, et al: Fluvoxamine treatment of social phobia (social anxiety disorder): a double-blind, placebo-controlled study. Am J Psychiatry 156:756–760, 1999

Strauss CC, Lahey BB, Frick P, et al: Peer social status of children with social anxiety disorders. J Consult Clin Psychol 56:137–141, 1988

Taylor S: Meta-analysis of cognitive-behavioral treatments for social phobia. J Behav Ther Exp Psychiatry 27:1–9, 1996

Turner SM, Beidel DC, Dancu CV, et al: An empirically derived inventory to measure social fears and anxiety: the Social Phobia and Anxiety Inventory. Psychol Assess 1:35–40, 1989

Van Ameringen M, Mancini C, Oakman JM: Nefazodone in social phobia. J Clin Psychiatry 60:96–100, 1999

Van Ameringen MA, Lane RM, Walker JR, et al: Sertraline treatment of generalized social phobia: a 20-week, double-blind, placebo-controlled study. Am J Psychiatry 158:275–281, 2001

van Vliet IM, den Boer JA, Westenberg HG, et al: Clinical effects of buspirone in social phobia: a double-blind placebo-controlled study. J Clin Psychiatry 58:164–168, 1997

Versiani M, Nardi AE, Mundim FD, et al: Pharmacotherapy of social phobia: a controlled study with moclobemide and phenelzine. Br J Psychiatry 161:353–360, 1992

Wallace ST, Alden LE: Social phobia and positive social events: the price of success. J Abnorm Psychol 106:416–424, 1997

Wells A, Papageorgiou C: Social phobia: effects of external attention on anxiety, negative beliefs, and perspective taking. Behav Ther 29:357–370, 1998

Wells A, Clark DM, Salkovskis P, et al: Social phobia: the role of in-situation safety behaviors in maintaining anxiety and negative beliefs. Behav Ther 26:153–161, 1995

Wolpe J: Psychotherapy by Reciprocal Inhibition. Stanford, CA, Stanford University Press, 1958

5

Obsessive-Compulsive Disorder

Brian Martis, M.D.
Nancy J. Keuthen, Ph.D.
Kimberly A. Wilson, Ph.D.
Michael Jenike, M.D.

Phenomenology

Symptoms

Obsessive-compulsive disorder (OCD) is characterized by obsessions and compulsions that intrude into a person's psychological and daily life by creating distress, taking inordinate periods of time, and increasing the risk of comorbidity, such as major depression. Obsessions are intrusive, disturbing, and incessant thoughts, ideas, images, or urges. Compulsions are repetitive mental or motor activities that mostly occur in response to obsessions and serve to neutralize anxiety. The compulsive acts themselves may have no clear relation to the obsessions (e.g., counting to a certain number to prevent harm) or are clearly excessive (e.g., washing countless times because one's hands "don't feel clean"). With some exceptions (in children and those with chronic poor insight), most patients are at least partially aware of the irrationality of their symptoms. Fear of contamination, pathological doubt, somatic obsessions, and need for symmetry are among the most common obsessions, whereas checking, washing, counting, the need to ask or confess, and symmetry/precision are among the more common compulsions. Most patients experience multiple obsessions and compulsions over time, though very rarely patients may have pure obsessions or compulsions (Table 5–1). A few recent studies using factor-analysis methods have identified symptom domains such as symmetry/hoarding, contamination/checking, and pure obsessions (Baer 1994), as well as obsessions/checking, symmetry/ordering, cleanliness/washing, and hoarding (Leckman et al. 1997), in an attempt to investigate clinically meaningful subtypes of OCD (Mataix-Cols et al. 1999). Symptom domains are considered to be somewhat stable over time, although the content of obsessions is known to change (Mataix-Cols et al. 2002).

Table 5–1.   Obsessive-compulsive symptoms on admission ($N=560$)

Obsessions	%	Compulsions	%
Contamination	50	Checking	61
Pathologic doubt	42	Washing	50
Somatic	33	Counting	36
Need for symmetry	32	Need to ask or confess	34
Aggressive	31	Symmetry and precision	28
Sexual	24	Hoarding	18
Multiple obsessions	72	Multiple compulsions	58

Source.   Eisen JL, Rasmussen SA: "Phenomenology of Obsessive-Compulsive Disorder," in *Textbook of Anxiety Disorders.* Edited by Stein DJ, Hollander E. Washington, DC, American Psychiatric Publishing, 2002, p. 179. Used with permission.

Patients are often secretive about their symptoms and suffering and are likely to present many years after the onset of the disorder (5–15 years, although this may change in light of increased awareness and treatment opportunities). Patients may be self-referred for OCD symptoms or may present with other clinical issues (e.g., separation anxiety, school refusal, or behavioral problems in children or adolescents; poor scholastic and/or work performance, depression, or substance abuse in adulthood). In women, onset or exacerbation of OCD during or after pregnancy has been noted. Often patients are first seen by a family physician, dermatologist, or practitioner of another medical subspecialty on the basis of their symptom presentation. As discussed below, obsessive-compulsive symptoms may also be present as manifestations of other neuropsychiatric disorders.

The DSM-IV-TR (American Psychiatric Association 2000) diagnostic criteria for OCD are presented in Table 5–2. It is important to be aware that many patients may not volunteer embarrassing or distressing symptoms (e.g., aggressive or sexual symptoms), and the risk of missing the diagnosis in this disorder despite characteristic symptoms is significant.

Associated Features

There is growing awareness of the extent to which OCD is associated with disability, including family dysfunction, as well as with a negative impact on quality of life. In one important study, OCD was found to be the tenth most disabling of all medical disorders (Murray and Lopez 1996).

Earlier retrospective studies of course of illness in adult OCD have consistently reported that the majority of people with OCD suffer a chronic course with some symptom fluctuations over time (assessed 2 or more years after diagnosis). However, these studies have been limited by methodological difficulties that often plague retrospective design, further confounded by the lack of standardized scales for comparison. More recent studies using rigorous methodology (such as reliable methods to standardize diagnosis and measure severity of symptoms), including a few prospective studies in younger and adult populations (with variable 2- to 7-year follow-up periods), generally confirm that approximately one-half to two-thirds of patients continue to fulfill the original diagnostic criteria at follow-up reevaluation (Flament et al. 1990; Leonard et al. 1993). Thus, patients with OCD may continue to have symptoms at varying levels of disability. Many of those considered improved continue to be in treatment, suggesting chronicity as well as the need for prolonged treatment for many OCD patients. A small percentage are considered to be in full or partial remission, although one-half of these patients have a subsequent relapse. Less than 15% are estimated to have an episodic course with partial or full remission, and in a small proportion of patients, the dis-

Table 5–2.   DSM-IV-TR diagnostic criteria for obsessive-compulsive disorder

A.   Either obsessions or compulsions:
Obsessions as defined by (1), (2), (3), and (4):
   (1)   recurrent and persistent thoughts, impulses, or images that are experienced, at some time during the disturbance, as intrusive and inappropriate and that cause marked anxiety or distress
   (2)   the thoughts, impulses, or images are not simply excessive worries about real-life problems
   (3)   the person attempts to ignore or suppress such thoughts, impulses, or images, or to neutralize them with some other thought or action
   (4)   the person recognizes that the obsessional thoughts, impulses, or images are a product of his or her own mind (not imposed from without as in thought insertion)
   Compulsions as defined by (1) and (2):
   (1)   repetitive behaviors (e.g., hand washing, ordering, checking) or mental acts (e.g., praying, counting, repeating words silently) that the person feels driven to perform in response to an obsession, or according to rules that must be applied rigidly
   (2)   the behaviors or mental acts are aimed at preventing or reducing distress or preventing some dreaded event or situation; however, these behaviors or mental acts either are not connected in a realistic way with what they are designed to neutralize or prevent or are clearly excessive
B.   At some point during the course of the disorder, the person has recognized that the obsessions or compulsions are excessive or unreasonable.   **Note:** This does not apply to children.
C.   The obsessions or compulsions cause marked distress, are time consuming (take more than 1 hour a day), or significantly interfere with the person's normal routine, occupational (or academic) functioning, or usual social activities or relationships.
D.   If another Axis I disorder is present, the content of the obsessions or compulsions is not restricted to it (e.g., preoccupation with food in the presence of an eating disorder; hair pulling in the presence of trichotillomania; concern with appearance in the presence of body dysmorphic disorder; preoccupation with drugs in the presence of a substance use disorder; preoccupation with having a serious illness in the presence of hypochondriasis; preoccupation with sexual urges or fantasies in the presence of a paraphilia; or guilty ruminations in the presence of major depressive disorder).
E.   The disturbance is not due to the direct physiological effects of a substance (e.g., a drug of abuse, a medication) or a general medical condition.

   Specify if:

      With Poor Insight: if, for most of the time during the current episode, the person does not recognize that the obsessions and compulsions are excessive or unreasonable order seems to follow a chronic deteriorating course. Sustained total remission of OCD is not usual.

Epidemiology

In contrast to the perception of OCD as a rare disorder in the mid-twentieth century, several recent epidemiological studies conducted in the United States and other parts of the world suggest that OCD is a fairly common disorder, with a lifetime prevalence of 2%–2.5% worldwide (Robins et al. 1984; Weissman et al. 1994). In the United States, this translates to approximately 5 million to 6 million Americans with clinical OCD. Unfortunately, the disorder continues to be undiagnosed or inappropriately treated, contributing to the enormous costs associated with OCD.

The onset of OCD is predominantly in childhood and young adulthood. In one study of 250 patients, the mean age at onset of OCD was reported to be 19.5±9.2 years in males versus 22±9.8 years in females ($P<0.003$), and 65% of patients experienced the onset of significant symptoms before age 25 years (less than 15% after age 35 years) (Rasmussen and Eisen 1998). In child and adolescent populations, studies have reported a predominance of males. In one such study of 70 subjects between ages 6 and 18 years, 47 (67%) were males, which may reflect an earlier onset of OCD in males (Leonard et al. 1989). Some cases of early-onset OCD may be characterized by an increase in specific symptoms clusters (sexual, aggressive, and symmetry obsessions and ordering and checking compulsions) and a history of tic-related symptoms. Earlier age of onset has also been reported to be associated with increased familial transmission of OCD (Pauls et al. 1995). In adult populations, OCD has been reported to be slightly more predominant in women than in men (Foa et al. 1995). Studies of marital status reveal that a significant number of people with OCD remain unmarried (43% in one study; Rasmussen and Eisen 1991). More research is required to understand the causative or prognostic implications of this finding.

Assessment

Obsessive-compulsive symptoms, when reported, are quite characteristic and hard to miss. However, patients are usually secretive about symptoms, so it is not uncommon that this diagnosis is missed in atypical presentations. OCD can present in childhood, adolescence, and adulthood. Childhood presentations may be disguised as presentations of separation anxiety, oppositional behavior, or school refusal. Similarly, adolescent OCD may present as depression, oppositional behavior, or scholastic difficulties. Adults are usually self-referred or referred by another clinician, and it is not unusual for some patients with OCD who are preoccupied with somatic concerns to visit primary care physicians, dermatologists, and physicians of other specialties. Obsessive-compulsive symptoms can also occur in other disorders such as schizophrenia, depression, tic-related disorders, and eating disorders. Very rarely, they may be the manifestations of an undiagnosed neurological disorder, such as a basal ganglia disorder or a vascular disorder. (Onset of illness de novo after age 45 years should trigger suspicion and a careful workup.) Four simple screening questions may help family physicians as well as psychiatric clinicians in busy practices screen for the presence of obsessive-compulsive symptomatology:

1. Do you have to wash your hands over and over?
2. Do you have to check things repeatedly?
3. Do you have thoughts that come into your mind that cause distress that you can't stop thinking about?
4. Do you need to complete actions over and over until they are just right or in a certain way before you can move on to the next thing?

A positive answer on any of these should be followed by a more careful evaluation for the presence of OCD (Rasmussen and Eisen 1997).

Comorbid disorders, which are not uncommon, may complicate therapeutic planning and must be looked for in every case of suspected OCD. Commonly present are depression, other anxiety disorders (panic disorder and social phobia), anorexia nervosa, schizophrenia, personality disorders, and alcohol abuse. It may also be wise not to diagnose personality disorder during an initial acute presentation of OCD, as some of these traits may resolve with treatment (Ricciardi et al. 1992). In a comprehensive interview, the clinician should also assess for variables that might impact treatment compliance or outcome, including overvalued ideation, secondary gain for obsessive-compulsive symptoms, and the nature of the home environment. A detailed treatment history specifically evaluating the nature of cognitive-behavioral therapy (CBT) received as well as medication trial adequacy is highly desirable. Finally, it is always important to assess past and present suicidality of patients with OCD.

Differential Diagnosis

Table 5–3 lists some common differential diagnoses that need to be considered when evaluating a suspected case of OCD. Comorbid disorders, including mood and other anxiety disorders and tic disorders, should be screened for, and in patients with comorbidity, an attempt should be made to determine the temporal sequence of symptoms. Careful, accurate diagnosis is critical for treatment planning and thus prognosis. For example, some studies suggest a less favorable prognosis for patients with comorbid schizotypal disorder or with a comorbid psychotic disorder. In the presence of psychotic symptoms, it is valuable to differentiate whether the patient has a comorbid, independent psychotic disorder (thus suggesting poorer prognosis and the need for an antipsychotic agent) or a single psychotic symptom of poor insight into his or her obsessions (in which case the patient may respond to medications similarly to the way an individual with good insight responds).

Assessment Measures

Assessment can be greatly enhanced by using adjunctive standardized instruments such as the Structured Clinical Interview for DSM-IV, Clinician Version (SCID-CV; First et al. 1996); obsessive-compulsive checklists and severity rating scales (such as the Yale-Brown Obsessive Compulsive Scale [YBOCS]; Goodman et al. 1989); and scales to measure depression (Beck Depression Inventory [BDI-II]; Beck et al. 1996), anxiety (Beck Anxiety Inventory [BAI]; Beck and Steer 1990), and other comorbid symptoms (tics, skin picking, hair pulling, etc.). Inclusion of simple assessments of clinical severity and work and social impact of OCD, such as the Clinical Global Impression (Guy 1976) and Work and Social Adjustment Scale (Mundt et al. 2002), may enhance clinical monitoring as well as aid in advocating effective treatment coverage for patients with their health insurance plan. Assessment packets can be individualized, depending on a clinic's particular clinical and research focus.

Pathogenesis

OCD is currently understood to include a group of heterogeneous conditions predominantly characterized by obsessions and compulsions. Although cau-

Table 5–3.   Differential diagnosis of obsessive-compulsive disorder

Axis I

With obsessive-compulsive features
1.   Major depressive disorder (with "obsessive" rumination)
2.   Delusional disorder (somatic obsessions)
3.   Body dysmorphic disorder
4.   Specific or social phobia
5.   Hypochondriasis
6.   Eating disorders
7.   Schizophrenia
8.   Other disorders with "compulsive" symptomatology (trichotillomania, paraphilias, pathological gambling, substance abuse)

With anxiety
1.   Panic disorder
2.   Posttraumatic stress disorder
3.   Generalized anxiety disorder

Axis II
1.   Pervasive developmental disorders
2.   Obsessive-compulsive personality disorder

Late onset (after 45 years)
Evaluate for neuromedical illness: history (especially family history and exposure to environmental toxins), neuroexamination, basic clinical workup, and neurodiagnostics as indicated
1.   Neurodegenerative (e.g., Huntington's chorea)
2.   Traumatic (rare anecdotal reports)
3.   Neoplastic and vascular

sation remains elusive, considerable progress has been made in advancing the understanding of various aspects of the mediation of these disorders.

Genetic Epidemiology

Findings from several rigorously conducted studies have supported the clinical and early research observations of the familial nature of OCD. First-degree relatives of probands with OCD (vs. healthy control subjects) tend to have a higher risk of developing clinical and subclinical OCD, more so when probands were younger at onset of OCD (<19 years old). Studies have also reported the association of OCD symptoms and OCD with tic disorders (including Tourette's disorder) and an overlapping familial pattern of these disorders (Pauls et al. 1986, 1995). On the basis of these and other studies, the existence of two familial forms of OCD has been suggested: a subgroup of OCD with early onset, associated with tic disorders and a non-tic-related presentation (see Wolff et al. 2000 for review). Current research involves the better characterization of the OCD subtypes and attempts to find consistent associated biogenetic markers of vulnerability.

Neuroanatomy

The long-standing clinical observations of obsessive-compulsive symptoms in certain conditions involving the basal ganglia (e.g., Sydenham's chorea), and more recent evidence from functional imaging studies in OCD, implicate the cortical (prefrontal)-striatal-thalamic-cortical pathways in the clinical manifestations of OCD. The findings from several resting-state functional neuroimaging studies demonstrate hyperactivity of the orbitofrontal cortex, anterior cingulate cortex, and, less consistently, the caudate nucleus. Serotonergic agents as well as exposure and response prevention (ERP) treatments have been shown to attenuate this hyperactivity (Baxter et al. 1996). Subtle deficits elicited by tests of frontostriatal functions have been demonstrated in patients with OCD. Neurosurgical interruption of certain neural pathways, including the frontothalamic pathways, has been shown to attenuate obsessive-compulsive symptoms in patients with severe OCD. These combined lines of evidence have resulted in corticostriatal models of the pathophysiology of OCD (see Rauch 2002 for review). One prevalent theory involves an imbalance in the direct and indirect corticostriatothalamic pathways that results in a net corticothalamic overdrive, postulated to result in characteristic symptoms of OCD. Certain putative subtypes of OCD, such as those marked by younger onset, male predominance, or comorbid tics or triggered by infection (PANDAS, pediatric autoimmune neuropsychiatric disorders associated with streptococcal infections; Swedo et al. 1998), may have specific associated etiologies.

Neurochemistry

The demonstration that clomipramine (CMI), a tricyclic antidepressant (TCA) with significant serotonergic effects, and later that selective serotonin reuptake inhibitors (SSRIs) attenuated OCD symptoms (independent of antidepressive effects), spurred much research into the serotonergic system in

OCD (Murphy et al. 1989; Zohar and Insel 1987). The reliance, due to inherent difficulties in studying the living human brain, on peripheral markers of central serotonergic functions (e.g., platelet 5-HT system and cerebrospinal fluid 5HIAA levels) has not shed meaningful light on pathogenesis. Functional neuroimaging studies currently under way promise a better way to study central serotonergic and other neurotransmitter systems. Thus, serotonergic modulation appears to partially affect OCD symptomatology. More recently, other systems have been implicated, such as the dopamine, glutamate, GABA (γ-aminobutyric acid), and neuropeptide systems (McDougle et al. 1999).

Management

Assessment and treatment of patients follow the general principles outlined in the introductory chapter on anxiety disorders (Chapter 1 in this volume). Treatment of OCD consists of educating the patient and family and outlining an individualized plan consisting of psychotherapy and/or pharmacotherapy in conjunction with other possibly required services (support, family intervention, specific addressing of school/vocational issues). Although each major component is separately discussed here, in reality, comprehensive treatment involves judicious concurrent use of all components. As previously noted, it is desirable to include objective parameters of symptoms, such as the YBOCS, in the initial assessment. While the YBOCS was designed as a clinician-rated instrument, patients can also be instructed in the use of the YBOCS as an inventory to monitor symptom severity. When the YBOCS is thus used, it is important for the clinician to review the patients' understanding of his or her obsessive-compulsive symptoms and the rating of each item (for example, items 5 and 9 concerning "resistance" may be confusing and need explanation). Such documentation helps greatly in capturing a baseline and the assessment of response. Additionally, third-party payers are increasingly adopting such ratings to determine eligibility for services.

A commonly encountered practical issue is one of payment for services. Health insurance plans and federal government plans vary regionally in the coverage they offer. Most plans approve one or more evaluation sessions. After making the diagnosis and initial treatment plan, the clinician usually has to seek approval for ERP and medication monitoring. A good strategy is to perform a thorough assessment, present the recommendations and various treatment alternatives to the patient, and work out a treatment strategy. The clinician can then advocate for standard-of-care services with the health plan.

Pharmacotherapy

Serotonin Reuptake Inhibitors

SSRIs are the usual first-line drugs for OCD (Expert Consensus Panel for Obsessive-Compulsive Disorder 1997). Table 5–4 lists the SSRIs used in the treatment of OCD, the recommended doses, and common side effects. It is important that patients be educated about the possible long response time (an adequate trial comprising 10–12 weeks), side effects, and alternatives. Anecdotally, it is sometimes noted that patients cannot tolerate even the lowest recommended doses, necessitating the use of even lower doses by either splitting tablets if possible or using liquid suspensions of these agents. This must always be anticipated and patients must always be educated about this possibility, as it could effect compliance.

Clomipramine is an effective antiobsessive that clinically has often taken second place because of its sometime troubling side effects. It is advisable to ensure a negative history of cardiac illness and do basic clinical tests, including a baseline electrocardiogram, before starting therapy with CMI. Occasionally, it may be useful to determine blood levels of CMI and its metabolite desmethyl-CMI (200–500 ng/mL) to guide treatment (especially during combination treatment with an SSRI), to investigate or prevent troubling side effects (less common but serious ones include risk of cardiac conduction delay and seizures), or in nonresponse.

There is increasing interest in venlafaxine for the treatment of OCD because of the similarity of its pharmacodynamic profile to that of CMI without the troublesome anticholinergic, antihistaminic, and α-adrenergic blocking effects. Findings from preliminary studies are encouraging (Albert et al. 2002), but controlled studies have yet to be completed.

Partial Response and Treatment Resistance

It is estimated that the symptoms of approximately 50% of patients with OCD respond partially to a trial with an SSRI. Consequently, a significant number of patients are left with residual symptoms and disability. Poor or

Table 5–4.   Pharmacotherapy of obsessive-compulsive disorder: first- and second-line medications, usual dose range, and common side effects

Drug	Usual dosing range[a] (effective range[b])	Duration of trial	Common significant side effects[c]	Remarks
Fluoxetine[d]	20–80 mg (40–80 mg)	12 weeks	Tremor, nervousness, insomnia, nausea, anorexia, delayed orgasm, asthenia Monitor for drug interactions related to cytochrome P450 2D6 inhibition. Significant drug interactions with TCAs (plasma levels of TCA ↑ 2–3-fold) Coadministration with MAOIs and thioridazine contraindicated	5 weeks' washout before MAOI Dose change frequency: one per week Prozac oral concentrate's strength is 4 mg/mL; the concentrate is mint flavored
Fluvoxamine (adults)[d]	50–300 mg (to 300 mg)	12 weeks	Tremor and nervousness, sleep disturbance, nausea, anorexia, delayed orgasm, asthenia Significant drug interactions with TCAs, warfarin, theophylline, propranolol, benzodiazepines Coadministration with MAOIs, pimozide, thioridazine, terfenadine, astemizole contraindicated	Split dose recommended if total exceeds 100 mg/day Dose change frequency: one every 3–4 days Lower doses in elderly patients and patients with hepatic impairment

Table 5–4. Pharmacotherapy of obsessive-compulsive disorder: first- and second-line medications, usual dose range, and common side effects (*continued*)

Drug	Usual dosing range[a] (effective range[b])	Duration of trial	Common significant side effects[c]	Remarks
Fluvoxamine[e]				
Age 8–11 years	25–200 mg	12 weeks	Agitation, hyperkinesia, decreased appetite and weight	Split dose recommended if total exceeds 50 mg/day
Age 11–18 years	25–200 mg (adolescents may require up to 300 mg)		Significant drug interactions with TCAs, warfarin, theophylline, propranolol, benzodiazepines	Dose change frequency: one every 3–4 days
			Coadministration with MAOIs, pimozide, thioridazine, terfenadine, astemizole contraindicated	Lower doses for children young than age 11 years (especially females)
Sertraline (adults)[d]	50–150 mg (to 200 mg)	12 weeks	Tremor and nervousness, dizziness, sleep disturbance, nausea, anorexia, delayed orgasm, asthenia	Once daily (morning or evening)
			Significant drug interactions with TCAs	Dosage change frequency: one per week
			Coadministration with MAOIs contraindicated	Lower doses in hepatic impairment

Table 5–4.   Pharmacotherapy of obsessive-compulsive disorder: first- and second-line medications, usual dose range, and common side effects (*continued*)

Drug	Usual dosing range[a] (effective range[b])	Duration of trial	Common significant side effects[c]	Remarks
Sertraline[e] Age 6–12 years Age 13–17 years	25–200 mg 50–200 mg	12 weeks	Nausea, agitation, insomnia, tremor, hyperkinesia, decreased appetite and weight Significant drug interactions with TCAs Coadministration with MAOIs contraindicated	Dose change frequency: one per week Lower dosages in low-body-weight children Zoloft oral concentrate's strength is 20 mg/mL, so concentrate must be diluted prior to administration; use contraindicated with disulfiram
Paroxetine	20–60 mg (40–60 mg)	12 weeks	Tremor, sleep disturbance, dry mouth, nausea, anorexia, constipation, sweating, abnormal ejaculation Monitor for drug interactions related to cytochrome P450 2D6 inhibition. Significant drug interactions with TCAs (plasma levels of TCA ↑ 2–3-fold) Coadministration with MAOIs and thioridazine contraindicated	Dosage change frequency: one per week Paxil oral concentrate's strength is 2 mg/mL; concentrate has orange flavor Caution in narrow-angle glaucoma

Table 5–4. Pharmacotherapy of obsessive-compulsive disorder: first- and second-line medications, usual dose range, and common side effects *(continued)*

Drug	Usual dosing range[a] (effective range[b])	Duration of trial	Common significant side effects[c]	Remarks
Clomipramine[d]	25–250 mg (up to 3 mg/ kg/day, to a maximum of 200 mg/day, in children and adolescents)	12 weeks	Dry mouth, constipation, urinary problems, postural hypotension, sedation and impaired concentration, weight gain, seizures Coadministration with most SSRIs results in 2–3-fold increase in plasma levels of clomipramine—caution! Coadministration with MAOIs contraindicated	Baseline cardiac and neurological history Baseline electrocardiogram recommended Blood levels of clomipramine and desmethyl-clomipramine recommended to guide clinician in certain clinical situations (e.g., troubling side effects, nonresponse, coadministration with SSRIs)

Note: MAOI = monoamine oxidase inhibitor; OCD = obsessive-compulsive disorder; SSRI = selective serotonin reuptake inhibitor; TCA = tricyclic antidepressant.

[a]Recommended dose ranges are based on manufacturers' package inserts (revised 2003).

[b]Effective dose ranges are based on the results of the few double-blind, placebo-controlled dose-range studies available.

[c]Information on side effects and drug interactions is adapted from results of double-blind, placebo-controlled trials and from manufacturers' package inserts and is *not* exhaustive. Side effect profiles are known to be different for the different SSRIs (even in the same patient), and side effects generally increase at higher doses. Clinicians are advised to be thoroughly familiar with the side effects and drug interactions of these medications before prescribing them, especially to special populations and in cases of polypharmacy.

[d]Approved by the U.S. Food and Drug Administration for acute treatment (10–13 weeks) of OCD in adults.

[e]Approved by the U.S. Food and Drug Administration for acute treatment of OCD (10 weeks) in children and adolescents.

nonresponse to first- and second-line agents should always trigger a review of diagnosis, comorbidity, compliance, and psychosocial stressors (especially family dynamics). Every attempt should be made to incorporate CBT early in the treatment algorithm.

If a patient's symptoms do not respond to one SSRI, the use of a different one within the class is usually recommended. If clinical circumstances permit, all available SSRI agents should be tried. Usually these drugs can be switched without significant difficulty. However, it is important to educate patients about discontinuation symptoms that may occur. Although SSRIs are relatively non-noxious, their effects on activity and sleep may require timely dosage, and potential sexual side effects should be anticipated and monitored in sexually active patients.

Some patients with OCD (with and without associated tics) who do not respond to an SSRI trial may respond upon addition of a low dose of a neuroleptic (e.g., haloperidol, risperidone) (McDougle et al. 1994, 2000). In cases of nonresponse to SSRIs or CMI, augmentation with several agents such as lithium, buspirone, pindolol, and amphetamines has been tried with variable success in some patients (Jenike et al. 1998). There is limited evidence for the use of MAOIs in OCD, but they could be considered in treatment-resistant OCD, especially when patients have predominant symmetry-related or other atypical obsessions, comorbid anxiety disorders, or atypical depression (Hollander et al. 2002). One experimental strategy being evaluated in nonresponders is intravenous bolus and pulse-loading of CMI; the results of two controlled studies are promising (Fallon et al. 1998; Koran et al. 1997).

Although the term *treatment resistance* has been used variably, it usually would include cases in which *at least* two SSRI trials, one CMI trial, and an adequate trial of ERP (approximately 20 hours) have failed. Such patients may be treated in a collaborative, carefully discussed stepwise manner, advancing from the best-studied to the less well studied strategies. It is important to involve the patient at every step of this process and document the rationale for off-label use of treatments. Early in this process, a consultation with a psychopharmacologist with expertise in OCD may prevent unnecessary suffering and expense for the patient and must be seriously considered. Figure 5–1 is a suggested algorithm for the treatment of newly diagnosed OCD, with extended strategies for treatment-refractory disease. It is important to carefully ascertain and document adequate treatment trials to prevent the patient's OCD from spuriously being labeled resistant. Chronic refractory OCD causing documented persistent, severe disability is sometimes treated palliatively with neurosurgical procedures such as anterior cingulotomy or anterior capsulotomy in specialized centers equipped to perform such interventions (Jenike et al. 1998).

Psychotherapy

ERP and the more recent cognitive therapy (CT) approaches are the two psychologically based treatments for OCD with some empirical documentation of efficacy. ERP was first developed in the 1960s, though not commonly used until the 1990s. Alternatively, CT is a much more recent, innovative approach with considerable promise of efficacy, although substantial outcome data for it are still lacking.

We discuss here both the behavioral and cognitive models for OCD and the specific treatment techniques that derive from each theoretical framework. Although we review the two models separately for the purposes of this chapter, we encourage clinicians to incorporate techniques from each approach in a coordinated fashion throughout the treatment process. Clinicians may occasionally find it necessary to begin treatment with cognitive techniques if patients refuse ERP. This is most likely to occur when they harbor intense fears of untoward outcomes on confronting their obsessions or when they are unable to tolerate the discomfort associated with ERP. In these cases, preliminary work with CT techniques may often enable the patient to subsequently engage in ERP.

Limited data currently exist addressing the relative benefits and costs of the behavioral and cognitive treatment approaches. As stated earlier, CT approaches still lack the wealth of empirical data that has accumulated over the years to validate the efficacy of ERP treatment. However, most experts anticipate that CT approaches will be beneficial and may, in certain situations, have some advantages over ERP. For example, it is reasonable to presume that lowered discomfort levels are associated with CT versus ERP because the former does not require direct confrontation of OCD triggers. In addition, it is also possible that CT is both more time- and cost-effective than ERP, though this hypothesis awaits rigorous examination. Until further research is available, we recommend that patients be offered treatments incorporating techniques from both approaches.

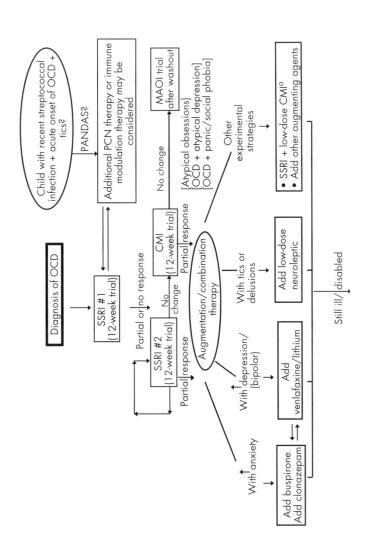

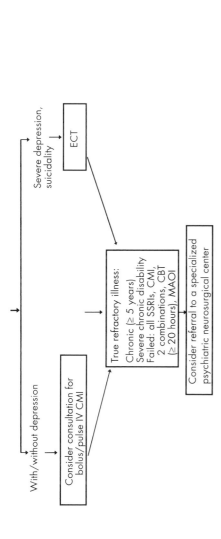

Figure 5–1. Suggested algorithm for medical management of obsessive-compulsive disorder. Every attempt should be made to incorporate cognitive-behavioral therapy early in the treatment algorithm.

CBT=cognitive-behavioral therapy; CMI=clomipramine; ECT=electroconvulsive therapy; IV=intravenous; MAOI=monoamine oxidase inhibitor; OCD= obsessive-compulsive disorder; PANDAS=pediatric autoimmune neuropsychiatric disorders associated with streptococcal infections; PCN=penicillin; SRI=serotonin reuptake inhibitor; SRI=selective serotonin reuptake inhibitor.

[a]Plasma levels of tricyclics may increase 2–10-fold when combined with SSRIs metabolized via the hepatic cytochrome P450-2D6 pathway (e.g., fluoxetine, paroxetine).

Source. Adapted from Goodman WK: "Pharmacotherapy of OCD," in *Textbook of Anxiety Disorders.* Edited by Stein DJ, Hollander E. Washington, DC, American Psychiatric Publishing, 2002, p. 220. Used with permission.

Trained cognitive-behavioral therapists can be located through the clinical directories and therapist referral services provided by the Obsessive-Compulsive Foundation (http://www.ocfoundation.org) and the Association for the Advancement of Behavior Therapy (http://www.aabt.org).

Behavioral Model of Obsessive-Compulsive Disorder

Effective use of ERP techniques necessitates a solid grasp of the behavioral model of OCD. Simply stated, the behavioral model maintains that 1) obsessions cause anxiety and discomfort and 2) compulsions and avoidance are maladaptive ways of reducing or avoiding these feelings. Furthermore, rituals or avoidance behavior are maintained over time through a process called *negative reinforcement.* This means that the future probability of specific behaviors under similar circumstances will increase if those behaviors are successful in reducing anxiety and discomfort.

To illustrate this point, let us use the example of the patient with OCD who is preoccupied with obsessions focused on the fear of contracting a deadly disease. In this scenario, if hand-washing rituals effectively reduce the anxiety stemming from the morbid illness fears, this individual is likely to hand-wash whenever she has illness obsessions in the future. Similarly, the patient with OCD who is distressed by harming thoughts while driving his car may redrive his route, check local newspapers or radio stations for hit-and-run accident reports, or seek reassurance from passengers. If these behaviors routinely reduce his discomfort, he is likely to repeat them whenever he experiences similar thoughts of harming others with his car. Thus, a self-perpetuating cycle develops in which the patient routinely engages in rituals and avoidance, these behaviors are reinforced by anxiety reduction, and the anxiety associated with the obsessions never lessens, being preemptively diminished by the rituals.

The theoretical foundation for the treatment intervention of ERP is the learning principle of habituation. *Habituation* refers to the reduction in negative emotional states accompanying prolonged, repetitive exposure to triggering stimuli. Over time, and with repeated exposure, the feared stimuli lose their ability to provoke discomfort. This occurs only if the individual does not engage in any behaviors designed to reduce anxiety, such as rituals or avoidance. Thus, if the individual with disease fears was repeatedly exposed to stimuli that triggered obsessive thoughts and was not allowed to hand-wash, one would predict lessening of her anxiety over time.

ERP, the mainstay of psychological treatment for OCD, was developed from these learning principles (for a review, see Abramowitz 1996, 1997). It involves the confrontation of one's obsessive cues (exposure) while simultaneously preventing the occurrence of rituals (response prevention). ERP practices are preferably conducted in real-life (in vivo or direct), although they can also be performed in imagination (imaginal) when the feared situations are not easily recreated.

Implementing Exposure and Response Prevention Treatment

Prior to undertaking behavioral treatment, it is necessary to compile a complete inventory of OCD symptoms. All rituals (both overt and covert), OCD triggers (e.g., specific situations, obsessional thoughts, images, or impulses), and avoidance behaviors must be identified. Completion of a functional analysis of behavior will outline the entire behavioral sequence, including the mechanisms by which symptoms are maintained. For example, the handwasher in our earlier example would reduce her anxiety by repeatedly washing. Similarly, the driving and checking rituals for our other patient would also serve to decrease his discomfort. Although initially there is usually a clear connection between the triggers and the ritualistic behavior, over time the rituals may generalize to other stimulus situations. For example, the patient may later also exhibit cleaning compulsions when upset or angry and not just when experiencing anxiety from contamination obsessions.

As mentioned earlier in the section on assessment, OCD symptoms can be identified through detailed clinician evaluations, coupled with patient symptom monitoring and self-report instruments (e.g., YBOCS severity and symptom checklist scales). Monitoring logs provide the therapist with a comprehensive symptom list; identify variables that trigger or exacerbate obsessive-compulsive symptoms; provide a baseline assessment of symptom severity, frequency, and duration; establish patient accountability to the treatment process; and can function to reduce symptoms through the process of *reactivity.* The latter term refers to the process whereby symptom reduction occurs simply through the course of recording its occurrence. Clinician interviews coupled with standardized scales can identify additional symptoms that patients fail to classify as OCD (including subtle avoidance behaviors and mental rituals), as well as comorbid disorders.

Hierarchies for ERP practices are constructed on completion of a comprehensive inventory of OCD symptoms. A pool of ERP tasks is developed with items varying along several dimensions, including proximity and duration of exposure to feared stimuli. For example, hierarchy items for the patient with disease fears could include walking down the main corridor of a hospital, eating in the hospital cafeteria, walking onto a medical ward, and visiting a hospitalized patient for 15 minutes. Overt behavioral rituals and covert mental rituals are prevented or limited, with graduated exposures to feared stimuli. Patients are asked to estimate anxiety levels associated with ERP tasks using the 100-point Subjective Units of Discomfort Scale (SUDS; Wolpe 1982), with 0 representing complete relaxation and 100 representing worst possible anxiety. Separate hierarchies are usually constructed for different symptom classes. Most hierarchies include 15–20 exposure tasks separated by increments of 5–10 SUDS units. Initial ERP homework tasks usually are selected so that SUDS scores are scaled in the 30–40 range.

Patients are instructed in routine practice of their ERP tasks, usually on a daily basis. Advancement to more difficult ERP tasks occurs when tasks reliably provoke significantly lower SUDS scores than when initially scaled. Considerable individual differences in habituation rates exist both between and within individuals (when multiple symptoms are present). A rule of thumb is for the patient to remain in the individual exposure practice until the SUDS level initially peaks and then diminishes to approximately 50% of maximal SUDS levels. The pacing of ERP practices is generally consensually negotiated between patient and therapist and is dependent on the patient's motivation and level of tolerance for discomfort. Initial demonstration of ERP practices by clinicians or lay coaches ("participant modeling") can facilitate the treatment, as can support provided by significant others. Throughout ERP treatment, patients are reminded that with this treatment approach, the rituals will wane before the obsessions do.

Imaginal exposures can be used in those cases in which either in vivo or direct exposure is difficult to arrange or in which this type of exposure does not sufficiently provoke and process specific fears. Similar to the process for other exposure practices, a hierarchy of imaginal scenes can be developed and taped for repeated home practice. When constructing these scenarios, it is imperative to use the patient's own description of the imagined scenes, including the patient's own thoughts, emotions, and physiological reactions. Patients should be instructed to imagine themselves in the scene rather than observing it from a distance. For example, if a patient fears contracting AIDS and repetitively hand-washes to reduce feared contamination by HIV, one possible scene would be the individual contracting AIDS after touching a hospital doorknob and neglecting to carefully wash. The patient would repeatedly listen to this taped scene until the SUDS levels noticeably decreased during each practice session, and over time until it no longer reliably elicited high SUDS levels on presentation.

Loop tapes can be effective for patients with specific obsessions, including blasphemous or immoral thoughts and unlucky numbers and words, and for those who engage in neutralizing or "undoing" mental rituals. In these cases, patients would tape themselves verbalizing their obsessions and repeatedly listen to a loop tape while focusing on their obsessional triggers and preventing mental rituals. For example, a woman with blasphemous thoughts of desiring sex with Christ would be instructed to tape and listen to her statement "I want to have intercourse with Christ. I would forsake my family if I knew I could be intimate with Jesus just once." She would be instructed to focus carefully on this statement without subvocalizing the mental ritual "Forgive me God. I am not worthy of being in your presence."

Possible Reasons for Poor Outcome With Exposure and Response Prevention Treatment

There are several potential causes for the failure of ERP treatment. If the patient's anxiety levels fail to habituate appropriately, the clinician should reevaluate for the presence of mental rituals or subtle avoidance during ERP practices. In other cases, anxiety may fail to habituate because of comorbid depression, requiring postponement of ERP treatment until the depression is effectively addressed. When treatment outcome is positive but the benefits fail to generalize to other similar situations, it may be necessary for the ERP treatment to be programmed using a broader range of situational cues.

In those cases in which the patient has difficulty sustaining treatment motivation, possible options are to involve significant others to reinforce progress or to make treatment progress more salient through regular comparison of baseline and current scale scores or symptom logs. In other scenarios, it may be necessary to slow down the pace of treatment if the individual is unwilling to tolerate high levels of anxiety. Lastly, analysis of the psychosocial context can identify inadvertent reinforcement for the patient's symptoms (e.g., the spouse always drives because the patient has harming obsessions when operating a motor vehicle).

Recent research has begun to demonstrate that CT may be a viable alternative or adjunct to ERP and medication for OCD. The fundamental approach in this therapy is to help patients identify, track, and challenge distorted thinking so as to reduce distress over obsessions and, ultimately, decrease the frequency of intrusions and compulsions. To understand the therapy, it is important first to know the model on which the treatment is based.

Cognitive Model of Obsessive-Compulsive Disorder

The application of CT to OCD stems from the finding that the experience and content of intrusive thoughts are not unique to those with OCD. In fact, approximately 90% of the general population can report having these types of thoughts, images, or impulses (Rachman and de Silva 1978). What, then, makes intrusive thoughts normal experiences in some and pathological obsessions in others? One element that seems to differ in people with OCD is the presence of specific types of interpretations or appraisals of their thoughts, such as "I must be perfectly certain" or "I'll be blamed for any harm" (Obsessive Compulsive Cognitions Working Group 2001). These appraisals make intrusions particularly distressing. Those interpretations and the negative affect that follows lead to attempts to neutralize, which are intended to make things right. These neutralization attempts, or compulsions, are reinforced by the subsequent absence of the feared outcome and reduction in anxiety. When intrusions inevitably reemerge, this chain of events will more likely recur because it has been strengthened through reinforcement. Moreover, intrusions will likely return with great frequency because of the increased attentional focus generated by the appraisal. See Salkovskis (1985, 1989) for a more comprehensive description of the model.

Consider this illustration. Many people even without OCD have the thought that germs are crawling all over an old dollar bill. This is a normal intrusion, and most are able to let that thought pass. However, if a person also believes that he is responsible for protecting others from even remote harm, overestimates risk, and perceives that uncertainty is intolerable, that initial thought will be especially upsetting. He may then feel compelled to engage in neutralization to rid himself of those upsetting feelings. Similarly, it is not uncommon to have unwanted sexual or blasphemous thoughts pop into one's mind. However, if those intrusions get filtered through beliefs that thinking is as bad as doing and that thoughts can be controlled, those intrusions will likely cause distress and urges to engage in compulsions. According to this model, then, it is not the presence of obsessions that lead to OCD but the appraisals of those thoughts that maintain the disorder.

Implementing Cognitive Therapy

Based on the cognitive model and the data that support it, CT is used to intervene at that critical point of thought appraisal by helping patients identify and challenge the distorted thoughts that fuel the cycle of OCD. As patients learn to consider alternate interpretations that are more accurate and benign, distress is reduced, as is the subsequent urge to neutralize. The goals, then, of CT are to develop strategies to challenge distorted thinking to reduce distress over obsessions and, thus, reduce frequency of obsessions and compulsions.

As in any effective treatment, good CT is conducted in the context of a trusting therapeutic relationship and is guided by a thoughtful and individualized case conceptualization. From the beginning, the therapist discusses the formulation directly with the patient to ensure that the understanding is correct, to provide education, and to model the collaborative approach that will be present throughout the work. The case conceptualization incorporates the patient's current OCD problems and related stressors and emphasizes ways in which his or her particular maladaptive cognitions contribute to the maintenance of the disorder. Patients are provided information about the types of cognitive domains that are typical of people with OCD and are directed to consider which might be personally relevant. These domains include overimportance of and control over thoughts, overestimation of threat, exaggerated perception of responsibility, perfectionism, and low tolerance for uncertainty.

A critical piece of the initial treatment involves interactively teaching the model and ensuring that the patient accepts the rationale for treatment. The patient's personal examples are used frequently in the discussion to highlight the individual significance of the model. The dialogue is conducted Socratically to incorporate the patient's feedback to design the most effective treatment plan. Throughout treatment, the model is consistently used as a reference point, to tie symptoms to a cognitive understanding of the problem and to guide decisions about subsequent interventions. As part of the model presentation, patients are educated about the commonness of intrusions and review a lengthy list of intrusions reported by people without OCD in research studies. This highlights again that it is not the intrusion itself but rather how the person perceives it that determines how he or she will feel and behave.

The format of CT sessions is structured and present-oriented. From the onset of treatment, patients are socialized to the structure, which includes joint agenda setting, mood check, homework assignments, homework review, building of cognitive intervention skills, summary of session highlights, and feedback. This structure lends organization to the work and ensures that important tasks are accomplished. The bulk of most sessions is spent on identification of distortions and skill building around challenging these thoughts.

Evaluation Strategies

Many of the strategies discussed here are derived from Wilhelm and Steketee's unpublished manual for CT for obsessive-compulsive disorder (S. Wilhelm, G. Steketee, "Cognitive Therapy for Obsessive-Compulsive Disorder," unpublished treatment manual, 2001). See also Steketee's (1999) published protocol for additional ideas on cognitive and behavioral approaches.

In CT, patients learn to challenge their thinking by gathering evidence to evaluate the accuracy of thoughts and testing predictions both in and between sessions. Thought records are used to facilitate this process. Patients first use the thought records to become accustomed to noticing automatic thoughts, then use them to challenge thoughts and bring that information to session.

For example, one common cognitive distortion is the belief that thinking is as bad as doing. This is particularly salient for patients with sexual obsessions. One intervention for the distress that this belief creates is called the continuum technique. Patients are asked to rate on a visual analogue scale from 0 ("most moral person ever") to 100 ("most immoral person ever") how immoral they are for having their thought. They are then asked how immoral such people as a drunk driver, someone who tortures animals, a murderer, a serial killer, and so on. These comparisons continue, and after each comparison, patients are asked to reevaluate their own immorality. Most frequently, the rating drops significantly, and patients are asked to reevaluate their distress and their urge to neutralize.

To address misestimation of threat, patients are taught a technique to reevaluate probability. They identify each step that would have to occur to lead to the feared outcome, estimate the probability of each point in the sequence, and then multiply those estimates together to arrive at the true estimate of risk. For example, a patient who fears she will spread AIDS to her partner by touching a discolored railing might produce the following list:

To lead to this outcome, someone HIV-positive would have to have been here (probability estimate = 1/4). If that's so, he would have to have touched the railing in that exact spot (1/10). If that's so, he would have to leave some fluid there (1/50). If that's so, the virus would have to still be alive when I touched it (1/2). If that's so, it would have to survive in the air while I drove home to my partner (1/10). If that's so, I would have to touch my partner with the exact spot that touched the railing (1/2). If that's so, it would have to survive the transfer (1/2). If that's so, the place I touched on my partner would have to be an open sore (1/10). If that's so, the virus must generate actual infection (9/10).

With the aid of a calculator, the product of the patient's estimates are then used to illustrate the final cumulative chance of the hypothesized sequence. Even using figures that are likely overestimates of each step, the result in this example is approximately 5 in 10 million. Another way to help patients reevaluate risk is to ask them if they are willing to place money on their prediction. If they say yes, press them to say how much—and then ask why not more.

Another technique, the advantages/disadvantages technique, is used to challenge the usefulness of holding on to a particular belief. For example, a patient may hold the belief that it is important to understand perfectly every element of what he has read in his introductory psychology textbook and thus spends hours reading and rereading each page. In this intervention, he would be asked to outline the benefits of holding this belief (e.g., it motivates him to try to learn more) and costs (e.g., it is time-consuming, the increased anxiety interferes with his ability to digest what he has read, it maintains his OCD, he gets frustrated by the whole process and never enjoys his work). The therapist may also Socratically challenge the validity of the benefit or benefits on the list, and the patient is then led to evaluate the lists taken together to generate a thought challenge to use the next time the irrational thought occurs to him.

Behavioral experiments can also be used to test the accuracy of interpretations. These exercises are framed as scientific attempts to gather evidence to prove or disprove hypotheses and generate alternate ideas. For example, if a patient is concerned that her thoughts will lead to harm befalling others, she may be asked to engage in a behavioral experiment to test whether thinking of a particular celebrity with a broken leg will lead to injury. She would then deliberately set aside time to visualize the celebrity with a minor injury and evaluate the consequences. Data gathered from this experiment can then be used to generate a rational response that she can use when the automatic thought next emerges.

Similarly, behavioral experiments can be used to test the common interpretation "I should try to control my thoughts." In the thought-suppression technique, a patient is instructed to try very hard to control her thoughts—that is, to rid her mind of the obsession—every other day. On the alternate days, she is told to freely allow the obsession to enter her mind. In both cases, she is to log the occurrence of the thought. She will likely notice an elevated frequency on the days in which she attempted to suppress the thought. If using the obsession as the manipulated thought is perceived as too distressing, this experiment can be conducted with the thought of a pink elephant, for example.

The above descriptions are simply examples of the multitudes of ways in which therapists can help their patients with OCD collect evidence to evaluate their distorted beliefs and try alternate ways of thinking. CT is a collaborative and creative endeavor in which patients learn to challenge appraisals of their obsessions in the hopes of reducing distress over them and ultimately reducing urges to neutralize. Initial evaluation of these and related methods is encouraging (Cottraux et al. 2001; Jones and Menzies et al. 1998; Krochmalik et al. 2001; McLean et al. 2001; van Oppen et al. 1995; Wilhelm 2000) and indicates that CT may be a useful alternative or adjunct to medication and exposure with response prevention.

Conclusion

OCD is an early-onset disorder that is challenging not only for patients and their families but also for clinicians. In most patients, OCD runs a chronic course, with variable disability. Newer treatments, specifically ERP and serotonergic agents, have helped significantly in symptom amelioration and possibly in improving the quality of life for many patients with OCD. Although research on many aspects of OCD has provided cause for hope, much work remains to be done to understand the pathophysiology of this syndrome and to provide significant relief to a majority of the sufferers. It is hoped that future advances can realistically address long-term symptom remission in patients with OCD.

Careful assessment of OCD, related symptoms, and comorbid conditions and an integrative treatment approach with a well-rationalized strategy that is individually tailored are essential. A careful psychosocial analysis of factors, including family involvement, that maintain and exacerbate symptoms is essential for effective treatment. Clinicians should be sensitive to the global effects of this disorder on a person's life and address these effects in treatment.

A successful treatment program seamlessly integrates pharmacological, psychological, and social interventions to produce the maximum benefit. This also includes working closely with patient advocacy groups such as the Obsessive-Compulsive Foundation that can provide patients and families with valuable information about resources. Patients often benefit vastly from support groups, educational sessions, and other socially empowering opportunities afforded by similar groups. Several options exist for patients whose disease responds poorly or not at all to first-line treatments; these must be pursued systematically. Experimental drug and behavioral strategies are also available for patients with resistant disease.

References

Abramowitz JS: Variants of exposure and response prevention in the treatment of obsessive-compulsive disorder: a meta-analysis. Behav Ther 27:583–600, 1996

Abramowitz JS: Effectiveness of psychological and pharmacological treatments for obsessive-compulsive disorder: a quantitative review. J Consult Clin Psychol 65:44–52, 1997

Albert U, Aguglia E, Maina G, et al: Venlafaxine versus clomipramine in the treatment of obsessive-compulsive disorder: a preliminary single-blind, 12-week, controlled study. J Clin Psychiatry 63:1004–1009, 2002

American Psychiatric Association: Diagnostic and Statistical Manual of Mental Disorders, 4th Edition, Text Revision. Washington, DC, American Psychiatric Association, 2000

Baer L: Factor analysis of symptom subtypes of obsessive compulsive disorder and their relation to personality and tic disorders. J Clin Psychiatry 55 (suppl):18–23, 1994

Baxter LR Jr, Saxena S, Brody AL, et al: Brain mediation of obsessive-compulsive disorder symptoms: evidence from functional brain imaging studies in the human and nonhuman primate. Semin Clin Neuropsychiatry 1:32–47, 1996

Beck AT, Steer RA: Beck Anxiety Inventory Manual. San Antonio, TX, Psychological Corporation, 1990

Beck AT, Steer RA, Brown GK: Manual for Beck Depression Inventory—II. San Antonio, TX, Psychological Corporation, 1996

Cottraux J, Note I, Yao SN, et al: A randomized controlled trial of cognitive therapy in obsessive-compulsive disorder. Psychother Psychosom 70:288–297, 2001

Eisen JL, Rasmussen SA: Phenomenology of obsessive compulsive disorder, in Textbook of Anxiety Disorders. Edited by Stein DJ, Hollander E. Washington, DC, American Psychiatric Publishing, 2002, pp 173–189

Expert Consensus Panel for Obsessive-Compulsive Disorder: Treatment of obsessive-compulsive disorder. J Clin Psychiatry 58 (suppl 4):2–72, 1997

Fallon BA, Liebowitz MR, Campeas R, et al: Intravenous clomipramine for obsessive-compulsive disorder refractory to oral clomipramine: a placebo-controlled study. Arch Gen Psychiatry 55:918–24, 1998

Fenton WS, McGlashan TH: The prognostic significance of obsessive-compulsive symptoms in schizophrenia. Am J Psychiatry 143:437–441, 1986

First MB, Spitzer RL, Gibbon M, et al: Structured Clinical Interview for DSM-IV Axis I Disorders, Clinician Version (SCID-CV). Washington, DC, American Psychiatric Press, 1996

Flament MF, Koby E, Rapoport JL, et al: Childhood obsessive-compulsive disorder: a prospective follow-up study. J Child Psychol Psychiatry 31:363–380, 1990

Foa EB, Kozak MJ: DSM-IV-TR field trial: obsessive compulsive disorder. Am J Psychiatry 152:90–96, 1995

Goodman WK: Pharmacotherapy of OCD, in Textbook of Anxiety Disorders. Edited by Stein DJ, Hollander E. Washington, DC, American Psychiatric Publishing, 2002, pp 207–219

Goodman WK, Price LH, Rasmussen SA, et al: The Yale-Brown Obsessive Compulsive Scale, I: development, use, and reliability. Arch Gen Psychiatry 46:1006–1011, 1989

Guy W: ECDEU Assessment Manual for Psychopharmacology, Revised (DHEW Publ No [ADM] 76–338). Rockville, MD, National Institute of Mental Health, 1976

Hollander E, Bienstock CA, Koran LM, et al: Refractory obsessive-compulsive disorder: state-of-the-art treatment. J Clin Psychiatry 63 (suppl)6:20–29, 2002

Jenike MA, Rauch SL, Baer L, et al: Neurosurgical treatment of obsessive-compulsive disorder, in Obsessive-Compulsive Disorders: Practical Management. Edited by Jenike MA, Baer L, Minichiello WE. St. Louis, MO, Mosby, 1998, pp 592–610

Jones MK, Menzies RG: Danger ideation reduction therapy for obsessive-compulsive washers: a controlled trial. Behav Res Ther 36:959–970, 1998

Koran LM, Sallee FR, Pallanti S: Rapid benefit of intravenous pulse loading of clomipramine in obsessive-compulsive disorder. Am J Psychiatry 154:396–401, 1997

Krochmalik A, Jones MK, Menzies RG: Danger Ideation Reduction Therapy (DIRT) for treatment-resistant compulsive washing. Behav Res Ther 39:897–912, 2001

Leckman JF, Grice DE, Boardman J, et al: Symptoms of obsessive-compulsive disorder. Am J Psychiatry 154:911–917, 1997

Leonard HL, Swedo SE, Rapoport JL, et al: Treatment of obsessive-compulsive disorder with clomipramine and desipramine in children and adolescents: a double-blind crossover comparison. Arch Gen Psychiatry 46:1088–1092, 1989

Leonard HL, Swedo SE, Lenane MC, et al: A 2- to 7-year follow-up study of 54 obsessive-compulsive children and adolescents. Arch Gen Psychiatry 50:429–439, 1993

Mataix-Cols D, Rauch SL, Manzo PA, et al: Use of factor-analyzed symptom dimensions to predict outcome with serotonin reuptake inhibitors and placebo in the treatment of obsessive-compulsive disorder. Am J Psychiatry 156:1409–1416, 1999

Mataix-Cols D, Rauch SL, Baer L, et al: Symptom stability in adult obsessive-compulsive disorder: data from a naturalistic two-year follow-up study. Am J Psychiatry 159:263–268, 2002

McDougle CJ, Goodman WK, Leckman JF, et al: Haloperidol addition in fluvoxamine-refractory obsessive-compulsive disorder: a double-blind, placebo-controlled study in patients with and without tics. Arch Gen Psychiatry 51:302–308, 1994

McDougle CJ, Barr LC, Goodman WK, et al: Possible role of neuropeptides in obsessive compulsive disorder. Psychoneuroendocrinology 24:1–24, 1999

McDougle CJ, Epperson CN, Pelton GH, et al: A double-blind, placebo-controlled study of risperidone addition in serotonin reuptake inhibitor–refractory obsessive-compulsive disorder. Arch Gen Psychiatry 57:794–801, 2000

McLean PD, Whittal ML, Thordarson DS, et al: Cognitive versus behavior therapy in the group treatment of obsessive-compulsive disorder. J Consult Clin Psychol 69:205–214, 2001

Mundt JC, Marks IM, Shear MK, et al: The Work and Social Adjustment Scale: a simple measure of impairment in functioning. Br J Psychiatry 180:461–464, 2002

Murphy DL, Zohar J, Benkelfat C, et al: Obsessive-compulsive disorder as a 5-HT subsystem–related behavioural disorder. Br J Psychiatry Suppl Dec(8):15–24, 1989

Murray CJL, Lopez AD (eds): The Global Burden of Disease: A Comprehensive Assessment of Mortality and Disability From Diseases, Injuries, and Risk Factors in 1990 and Projected to 2020 (Global Burden of Disease and Injury, Vol 1). Cambridge, MA, Harvard University Press, 1996

Obsessive Compulsive Cognitions Working Group: Development and initial validation of the Obsessive Beliefs Questionnaire and the Interpretation of Intrusions Inventory. Behav Res Ther 39:987–1006, 2001

Pauls DL, Towbin KE, Leckman JF, et al: Gilles de la Tourette's syndrome and obsessive-compulsive disorder: evidence supporting a genetic relationship. Arch Gen Psychiatry 43:1180–1182, 1986

Pauls DL, Alsobrook JP 2nd, Goodman W, et al: A family study of obsessive-compulsive disorder. Am J Psychiatry 152:76–84, 1995

Rachman S, de Silva P: Abnormal and normal obsessions. Behav Res Ther 16:233–238, 1978

Rasmussen SA, Eisen JL: Phenomenology of obsessive-compulsive disorder, in Psycho-biology of Obsessive-Compulsive Disorder. Edited by Insel TJ, Rasmussen SA. New York, Springer-Verlag, 1991, pp 743–758

Rasmussen SA, Eisen JL: Treatment strategies for chronic and refractory obsessive-compulsive disorder. J Clin Psychiatry 58 (suppl 13):9–13, 1997

Rasmussen SA, Eisen JL: The epidemiology and clinical features of obsessive-compulsive disorder, in Obsessive-Compulsive Disorders: Practical Management, 3rd Edition. Edited by Jenike MA, Baer L, Minichiello WE. St. Louis, MO, Mosby, 1998, pp 12–43

Rauch SL, Cora-Locatelli G, Greenberg BD: Pathogenesis of obsessive-compulsive disorder, in Textbook of Anxiety Disorders. Edited by Stein DJ, Hollander E. Washington, DC, American Psychiatric Publishing, 2002, pp 191–205

Ricciardi JN, Baer L, Jenike MA, et al: Changes in DSM-III-R axis II diagnoses following treatment of obsessive-compulsive disorder. Am J Psychiatry 149:829–831, 1992

Robins LN, Helzer JE, Weissman MM, et al: Lifetime prevalence of specific psychiatric disorders in three sites. Arch Gen Psychiatry 41:949–958, 1984

Salkovskis P: Obsessional-compulsive problems: a cognitive-behavioural analysis. Behav Res Ther 23:571–583, 1985

Salkovskis P: Cognitive-behavioural factors and the persistence of intrusive thoughts in obsessional problems. Behav Res Ther 27:677–682, 1989

Steketee G: Overcoming Obsessive-Compulsive Disorder: A Behavioral and Cognitive Protocol for the Treatment of OCD—Therapist Protocol. Oakland, CA, New Harbinger Publications, 1999

Swedo SE, Leonard HL, Garvey M, et al: Pediatric autoimmune neuropsychiatric disorders associated with streptococcal infections: clinical description of the first 50 cases. Am J Psychiatry 155:264–271, 1998

van Oppen P, de Haan E, van Balkom A, et al: Cognitive therapy and exposure in vivo in the treatment of obsessive compulsive disorder. Behav Res Ther 33:379–390, 1995

Weissman MM, Bland RC, Canino GJ, et al: The cross-national epidemiology of obsessive compulsive disorder. The Cross-National Collaborative Group. J Clin Psychiatry 55 (suppl):5–10, 1994

Wilhelm S: Cognitive therapy for obsessive-compulsive disorder. J Cognit Psychother 14:245–259, 2000

Wolff M, Alsobrook JP 2nd, Pauls DL: Genetic aspects of obsessive-compulsive disorder. Psychiatr Clin North Am 23:535–544, 2000

Wolpe J: The Practice of Behavior Therapy, 3rd Edition. Oxford, UK, Pergamon, 1982

Zohar J, Insel TR: Obsessive-compulsive disorder: psychobiological approaches to diagnosis, treatment, and pathophysiology. Biol Psychiatry 22:667–687, 1987

6

Posttraumatic Stress Disorder and Acute Stress Disorder

Randall D. Marshall, M.D.

Barbara Rothbaum, Ph.D.

Phenomenology

Symptoms

Although described for centuries, the existence of a universal posttraumatic syndrome was not officially acknowledged until 1980, by DSM-III (American Psychiatric Association 1980), and much has been said about the politics and social bias of this resistance to recognizing such a clinically disabling syndrome (Herman 1992). The delineation of a posttraumatic stress syndrome (PTSD) in both the U.S. and international diagnostic manuals subsequently facilitated worldwide research on symptoms, epidemiology, disability, and treatment for those who have the disorder.

One of the primary confusions in the literature, and among health professionals, is distinguishing between trauma and stress. Both have been associated with a wide range of psychological and medical disabilities, and both can be a source of severe anxiety. DSM-IV-TR (American Psychiatric Association 2000) defines trauma (Criterion A for PTSD) as an event in which "the person experienced, witnessed, or was confronted with an event or events that involved actual or threatened death or serious injury, or a threat to the physical integrity of self or others; [and] the person's response involved intense fear, helplessness, or horror. In children, this may be expressed instead by disorganized or agitated behavior." It is very important for clinicians working with children to note that "for children, sexually traumatic events may include developmentally inappropriate sexual experiences without threatened or actual violence or injury." The consequences of these kinds of experiences are qualitatively different from those of stressors such as job loss, divorce, poverty, and social isolation (Kendler et al. 1999), which in general are most strongly associated with major depression. and which are not causes of PTSD.

A wide range of fairly common experiences fall within this definition of trauma, such as car accidents, industrial accidents, experiences of domestic violence, robbery, criminal assault, rape, natural disasters, and of course war-related experiences. Large epidemiological studies have shown that more than 60.7% of men and 51.2% of women in the United States and more than 50% of the adult community in Australia, for example, have experienced at least one such trauma (Australian Bureau of Statistics 1998; Kessler et al. 1995). The majority of individuals appear to recover from traumatic experiences without developing PTSD. It should also be kept in mind that PTSD is not the only outcome after traumatic events. Major depressive disorder, for example, is also common (Kendler et al. 1999; Shalev et al. 1998).

Large multicenter field trials have identified core features of posttraumatic reactions. These core features, as defined in DSM-IV-TR, are shown in the diagnostic criteria set in Table 6–1. For the clinician, they may be conceptualized as 1) vividly remembering the event in the form of thoughts, images, and dreams, with concomitant physiological reaction to these memories or reminders of the trauma; 2) persistent internal (psychological) and/or external (behavioral) avoidance of reminders of the trauma; 3) loss of interest in activities and detachment from others, a restricted range of affect (to mostly negative-valence emotions), and a sense of a foreshortened future; and 4) signs of chronically heightened sympathetic arousal, including both cognitive and physiological manifestations.

Table 6–1.   DSM-IV-TR diagnostic criteria for posttraumatic stress disorder

A. The person has been exposed to a traumatic event in which both of the following were present:
  (1) the person experienced, witnessed, or was confronted with an event or events that involved actual or threatened death or serious injury, or a threat to the physical integrity of self or others
  (2) the person's response involved intense fear, helplessness, or horror. **Note:** In children, this may be expressed instead by disorganized or agitated behavior
B. The traumatic event is persistently reexperienced in one (or more) of the following ways:
  (1) recurrent and intrusive distressing recollections of the event, including images, thoughts, or perceptions.   **Note:** In young children, repetitive play may occur in which themes or aspects of the trauma are expressed.
  (2) recurrent distressing dreams of the event.   **Note:** In children, there may be frightening dreams without recognizable content.
  (3) acting or feeling as if the traumatic event were recurring (includes a sense of reliving the experience, illusions, hallucinations, and dissociative flashback episodes, including those that occur on awakening or when intoxicated).   **Note:** In young children, trauma-specific reenactment may occur.
  (4) intense psychological distress at exposure to internal or external cues that symbolize or resemble an aspect of the traumatic event
  (5) physiological reactivity on exposure to internal or external cues that symbolize or resemble an aspect of the traumatic event
C. Persistent avoidance of stimuli associated with the trauma and numbing of general responsiveness (not present before the trauma), as indicated by three (or more) of the following:
  (1) efforts to avoid thoughts, feelings, or conversations associated with the trauma
  (2) efforts to avoid activities, places, or people that arouse recollections of the trauma
  (3) inability to recall an important aspect of the trauma
  (4) markedly diminished interest or participation in significant activities
  (5) feeling of detachment or estrangement from others
  (6) restricted range of affect (e.g., unable to have loving feelings)
  (7) sense of a foreshortened future (e.g., does not expect to have a career, marriage, children, or a normal life span)

Table 6–1.   DSM-IV-TR diagnostic criteria for posttraumatic stress disorder *(continued)*

D.   Persistent symptoms of increased arousal (not present before the trauma), as indicated by two (or more) of the following:
  (1)   difficulty falling or staying asleep
  (2)   irritability or outbursts of anger
  (3)   difficulty concentrating
  (4)   hypervigilance
  (5)   exaggerated startle response
E.   Duration of the disturbance (symptoms in Criteria B, C, and D) is more than 1 month.
F.   The disturbance causes clinically significant distress or impairment in social, occupational, or other important areas of functioning.

Specify if:
  Acute: if duration of symptoms is less than 3 months
  Chronic: if duration of symptoms is 3 months or more

Specify if:
  With Delayed Onset: if onset of symptoms is at least 6 months after the stressor

Trauma-related diagnoses are still under active scientific study, and there is still debate as to whether a syndromal, dimensional, or spectrum model provides the best fit for the clinical and etiological data available to date. It is clear that individuals with "subthreshold" symptoms (i.e., those with some symptoms but not meeting full criteria) also have some disability and might benefit from treatment (Marshall et al. 1999; Stein et al. 1997). The clinician would be wise therefore to be able to recognize the primary features of PTSD without being too wedded to the current syndromal definitions (Table 6–1).

Investigators also are debating whether the new diagnosis of acute stress disorder (ASD) is valid. Nevertheless, defining some version of an acute post-traumatic response syndrome is important in view of the possibility that particular kinds of early intervention may prevent the development of PTSD.

Associated Features

Numerous studies have demonstrated a high degree of global impairment and disability in PTSD, including work-related impairment (Blanchard et al. 1998), somatic complaints (McFarlane et al. 1994), lower quality of life (Cordova et al. 1995), suicidality (Davidson et al. 1991), medical illness (McFarlane et al. 1994), negative body image (Wenninger and Heiman 1998), impaired intimacy (Riggs et al. 1998), increased burden to spouse or partner (Beckham et al. 1996), and social dysfunction (Blanchard et al. 1998).

Adults with PTSD due to childhood trauma also appear to have higher rates of interpersonal problems and difficulties regulating affect compared with those experiencing other types of trauma (Cloitre et al. 1997).

Acute Stress Disorder

In DSM-III-R (American Psychiatric Association 1987), there was no diagnosis to capture PTSD-like symptoms in the first 30 days after a trauma. Because of concern about confounding normative reactions to trauma with pathological responses in this early phase, it was decided to create an acute diagnosis with relatively high specificity that might predict chronic PTSD. At the time, peritraumatic dissociation had been identified as an early clinical predictor of chronic disorder, and so the diagnosis of acute stress disorder was defined as requiring the three core symptom clusters plus three of five dissociative symptoms (Table 6–2).

Further empirical and theoretical work revealed significant problems with the diagnosis. (For reviews, see Harvey and Bryant 2002 and Marshall et al. 1999.) Most importantly, a significant proportion of people not meeting ASD criteria still developed chronic PTSD. In other words, the diagnosis has unacceptably low sensitivity either as a research tool or a diagnosis that permits access to care.

Epidemiology

PTSD is a serious, relatively common, often chronic illness, the study of which is of increasing importance to public health. The National Comorbidity Survey found a lifetime prevalence of PTSD of 10.4% for women and 5.0% for men in the United States (Kessler et al. 1995). Few data are available from war-ravaged nations and the developing world, where rates are possibly much higher. A number of vulnerability factors have been identified, including neuroticism, personality disorder, history of psychiatric illness, history of trauma or stress, genetic liability, and family history of psychiatric disorder (Yehuda 2002). These factors, however, are neither necessary nor sufficient to explain the presence of PTSD; thus, an assessment to ascertain the nature of the traumatic experience is still essential to making the diagnosis.

Table 6–2. DSM-IV-TR diagnostic criteria for acute stress disorder

A. The person has been exposed to a traumatic event in which both of the following were present:
  (1) the person experienced, witnessed, or was confronted with an event or events that involved actual or threatened death or serious injury, or a threat to the physical integrity of self or others
  (2) the person's response involved intense fear, helplessness, or horror
B. Either while experiencing or after experiencing the distressing event, the individual has three (or more) of the following dissociative symptoms:
  (1) a subjective sense of numbing, detachment, or absence of emotional responsiveness
  (2) a reduction in awareness of his or her surroundings (e.g., "being in a daze")
  (3) derealization
  (4) depersonalization
  (5) dissociative amnesia (i.e., inability to recall an important aspect of the trauma)
C. The traumatic event is persistently reexperienced in at least one of the following ways: recurrent images, thoughts, dreams, illusions, flashback episodes, or a sense of reliving the experience; or distress on exposure to reminders of the traumatic event.
D. Marked avoidance of stimuli that arouse recollections of the trauma (e.g., thoughts, feelings, conversations, activities, places, people).
E. Marked symptoms of anxiety or increased arousal (e.g., difficulty sleeping, irritability, poor concentration, hypervigilance, exaggerated startle response, motor restlessness).
F. The disturbance causes clinically significant distress or impairment in social, occupational, or other important areas of functioning or impairs the individual's ability to pursue some necessary task, such as obtaining necessary assistance or mobilizing personal resources by telling family members about the traumatic experience.
G. The disturbance lasts for a minimum of 2 days and a maximum of 4 weeks and occurs within 4 weeks of the traumatic event.
H. The disturbance is not due to the direct physiological effects of a substance (e.g., a drug of abuse, a medication) or a general medical condition, is not better accounted for by brief psychotic disorder, and is not merely an exacerbation of a preexisting Axis I or Axis II disorder.

Assessment

PTSD symptoms themselves are rarely the only source of difficulty in the patient's life, and a comprehensive psychiatric history and interview are needed to also assess other psychopathology (e.g., depression, panic attacks, personality disorder), social functioning (e.g., work and friendships), and issues of intimacy (e.g., family life).

Differential Diagnosis

Although the symptoms of PTSD overlap with a broad range of different psychiatric disorders, their specific association with a prior trauma is defining for PTSD. Clinical and epidemiological studies have shown that a history of trauma and symptoms of PTSD are usually missed, misdiagnosed, or inadequately addressed in both general medical and psychiatric settings (Eilenberg et al. 1996; Jacobson et al. 1987). This is probably because of several factors, including the patient's lack of awareness that his or her symptoms and problems are related to a traumatic experience, what it is that he or she feels permitted to seek help for (as opposed to having to overcome through individual effort), and the diagnostic skills of the clinician. For example, a victim of domestic violence may complain repeatedly about insomnia, diffuse somatic aches and pains, and depression—without ever mentioning her history of abuse to the physician.

Assessment Measures

Epidemiological surveys have shown that PTSD is rarely detected unless the individual is first asked about specific Criterion A traumas. One efficient way of doing this is by using a self-report questionnaire to assess life history of traumatic events. Perhaps the most widely used is the Life Stressor Checklist—Revised (Wolfe and Kimerling 1997). Once a trauma history has been identified, the response to the trauma can be assessed clinically and with one of a number of different rating scales. The rating scale currently used in most pharmacotherapy trials of PTSD is the Clinician-Administered PTSD Scale (CAPS; Blake et al. 1995), which has the additional advantage of clearly described questions and anchor points to assist with diagnosis (obtainable at http://www.ncptsd.org).

Pathogenesis

Alterations in multiple biological systems have been identified in both adults and children with PTSD. This is not surprising, because PTSD has the highest rate of comorbidity of any Axis I disorder and the most extensive overlap across the affective, anxiety, and personality disorders. Most biological findings remain controversial at present because of mixed results across research centers and subject populations. Although there are a number of explanatory models under development by various centers, all efforts are in their infancy.

A low-normal baseline cortisol level is one of the most widely replicated findings, though its endocrine pattern is not specific to PTSD. (For reviews, see Heim et al. 2000 and Yehuda 2002.) Perhaps the most consistent finding in chronic PTSD has been enhanced suppression of cortisol in response to low-dose dexamethasone. This suppression suggests a supersensitivity of the hypothalamic-pituitary-adrenocortical (HPA) axis and has been characterized as heightened negative feedback, perhaps at the receptor level (Yehuda 2002). Recent studies (e.g., Delahanty et al. 2000) suggest that HPA axis alterations are a preexisting characteristic of patients with PTSD and thus not due to the pathology itself. This is of particular interest both because it runs counter to traditional models of HPA axis functioning in response to stress and because it is the opposite of the primary HPA axis finding in major depression. In major depression, at a least a subgroup of patients have elevated cortisol levels and relative nonsuppression of cortisol on the dexamethasone test.

Findings have been more difficult to interpret in the catecholamine system. Adults with PTSD have consistently shown elevated heart rate and skin conduction in response to trauma-related cues. Findings of catecholamine functioning at baseline, however, have been mixed, with studies showing elevated, normative, or low levels of catecholamines and their metabolites.

Several studies have found reduced hippocampal volume in patients with PTSD compared with control subjects, but it was unknown whether this was a preexisting condition in these patients. (For review, see Hull 2002.) In an elegantly designed twin study, Pitman et al. (2002) recently confirmed the finding of reduced hippocampal volume in subjects with chronic PTSD but also showed that it was probably a preexisting condition and not a consequence of psychopathology. In monozygotic twin pairs in which only one twin had been exposed to severe trauma, PTSD severity in the exposed twin was negatively correlated with hippocampal size in the unexposed twin.

Imaging studies of PTSD are in their infancy, and the heterogeneity of the disorder makes comparisons across these small studies difficult, placing all the more importance on replication as a measure of validity for any finding. A general consensus is emerging on several findings and methodological issues, including 1) the importance of symptom-provocation paradigms in functional imaging studies; 2) the finding of hippocampal volumetric reduction; and 3) amygdala activation, reflecting the role of emotional memory in PTSD. It is unlikely that any of these findings is specific to PTSD; identification of common biological findings across psychiatric disorders is a relatively new priority in studies of the biological substrate of affective and anxiety-spectrum illness.

Neurocircuitry correlates of PTSD most likely involve multiple cortical and subcortical systems related to regulation of mood, memory, threat, circadian rhythms, and neuroendocrine function. Given the complexity of symptoms and the fact that the manifestations of PTSD occur in multiple domains, it is unlikely that a single circuit or brain locus is the primary alteration in brain function. It is also likely that it is a heterogeneous syndrome, meaning that there are probably multiple pathways and multiple alterations involved, all of which may manifest in some combination of PTSD symptoms.

Brain imaging technology is, however, on the verge of being able to investigate such complex patterns, and it is hoped that the immediate future will yield important findings in PTSD and many other disorders (reviewed in Grossman et al. 2002). An early example of imaging findings illustrates the complexity of such studies. Rauch et al. (1996) performed positron emission tomography scans with script-driven imagery in eight patients with PTSD screened as physiologically responsive to the imagery symptom provocation paradigm. Most (seven of eight) had suffered non-combat-related trauma. During exposure to audiotaped traumatic scripts, increases in blood flow were found in right-sided limbic, paralimbic, and visual areas; decreases were found in the left inferior frontal (Broca's area) and middle temporal cortex. There was no significant change within the hypothalamus, and there were increases in the right limbic and paralimbic structures, including posterior medial orbitofrontal, insula, anterior temporal, medial temporal, and anterior cingulate cortex, as well as the amygdala. The authors concluded that emotions associated with the PTSD symptomatic state may be mediated by the limbic and paralimbic systems in the right hemisphere. Visual cortex activation may correspond to the visual component of PTSD.

Serotonergic pathways project extensively throughout the brain, and to a number of areas that may be relevant to PTSD symptoms. Serotonin cell bodies are clustered in the pons and upper brain stem, and projections to the amygdala, hippocampus, and locus coeruleus may be relevant to the observed benefit of serotonergic medications discussed in the next section. Increased locus coeruleus activity over time may alter synaptic networks and result in perpetually elevated sympathetic responsivity. The locus coeruleus pathways to the hippocampus and amygdala may explain associated phenomena such as nightmares, flashbacks, and the repetitive perception of threat triggered by relatively innocuous stimuli.

Pharmacotherapy

Acute Stress Disorder

There are no controlled medication trials specifically for ASD. A nonrandomized trial of propranolol in people who had been acutely traumatized (only a minority of which would meet criteria for ASD) showed promising preliminary results (Vaiva et al., in press), but the first controlled trial of propranolol in adults experiencing severe trauma found minimal benefit for this drug as prophylaxis against developing PTSD (Pitman et al. 2002). Theoretically, reducing catecholaminergic activation in the acute setting might decrease risk for development of chronic disorder by blocking consolidation of the memory with fear networks, and future research will likely focus on this promising hypothesis.

Posttraumatic Stress Disorder

This chapter emphasizes results of controlled trials in adults with chronic PTSD. Most studies included patients who had been ill for many years, and the studies reported since the 1990s also deliberately included patients with comorbidity such as major depression, panic disorder, and social phobia. Most trials, however, do not include people with concurrent substance abuse problems, despite the fact that this is very common in PTSD. This is because it is considered unethical to include such patients without providing a treatment that addresses the substance use, yet to provide such treatment would compromise the study design. The best way to study this comorbidity is to focus specifically on this population, as many centers are doing at present.

Selective Serotonin Reuptake Inhibitors

Recent multicenter trials have shown that selective serotonin reuptake inhibitors (SSRIs) are effective in reducing PTSD symptoms both during acute treatment (Brady et al. 2000; Davidson et al. 2001b; Marshall et al. 2001a) and over an extended period of treatment (Londburg et al. 2001). There have been large multicenter trials for sertraline and paroxetine, and both are approved by the U.S. Food and Drug Administration (FDA) as a treatment for adults with PTSD.

Brady et al. (2000) reported that the first 12-week multicenter, placebo-controlled, randomized trial included a 1-week placebo run-in involving mostly subjects with non-combat-related trauma. The dropout rate was relatively low, at 54 of 187 subjects. In the intent-to-treat analysis, the response rate for sertraline was 53%, compared with 32% for placebo, when response was defined as "much improved" or "very much improved" on the Clinical Global Impression Scale (CGI) plus at least a 30% reduction in symptom severity on the CAPS. There was significant improvement in the symptom clusters of hyperarousal and avoidance but not of reexperiencing. Secondary measures showed improved quality of life and social and occupational function. Mean dosage was 151 mg/day at endpoint.

Davidson et al. (2001b) reported a second 12-week, multicenter, placebo-controlled, randomized trial of flexible-dosage sertraline ($n=100$) versus placebo ($n=108$) in adults (mostly women) with mixed trauma and chronic PTSD. All subjects had duration of illness of 6 months or more and baseline CAPS scores higher than 50. The intent-to-treat analysis found a 60% response rate for sertraline versus 38% for placebo ($P=0.004$). Patients taking sertraline experienced a 44.6% reduction in symptoms, compared with a 35% reduction in symptoms for those taking placebo. Most responders met the response criteria by week 4. The discontinuation rate was 11% for sertraline because of adverse events, compared with 5% for placebo. Sertraline was not superior to placebo on measures of depression, general anxiety, or sleep problems. In terms of individual symptom clusters, sertraline significantly reduced avoidance/numbing symptoms but neither reexperiencing nor hyperarousal as assessed by the CAPS (physician-rated). By self-report on the Davidson Trauma Scale, however, all three symptom clusters were reduced.

A third trial that also recruited primarily individuals with non-combat-related PTSD did not find sertraline to be superior to placebo (Physicians' Desk Reference 2001). Findings of a fourth trial also were negative, but the study was conducted primarily among male U.S. war veterans (Physicians' Desk Reference 2001).

In the study of Brady et al. (2000), sertraline was superior to placebo as assessed by CGI responder rates of 53% (sertraline) versus 32% (placebo). Overall, reductions in CAPS scores were from 76 to 43 for sertraline and from

75 to 52 for placebo. Sertraline was significantly superior to placebo in reducing the hyperarousal and avoidance clusters but not the reexperiencing cluster. The mean score (which includes both responders and nonresponders) after treatment with sertraline was still 43, a moderately symptomatic score.

A recent fixed-dose trial of paroxetine (Marshall et al. 2001a) randomly assigned patients to receive either 20 mg/day of paroxetine, 40 mg/day of paroxetine (achieved with gradual dosage increases), or placebo. Response rates (determined by CGI scores of 2 or 1), which were superior to placebo for both active treatment groups, were as follows: 63% for 20 mg/day paroxetine, 57% for 40 mg/day paroxetine, and 37% for placebo. Reduction in CAPS scores were as follows: 75.3–35.7 for 20 mg/day paroxetine, 74.3–36.4 for 40 mg/day paroxetine, and 74.4–49.1 for placebo. This was the first SSRI study to demonstrate efficacy in all three clusters of PTSD symptoms. Paroxetine was superior to placebo in both males and females, a finding also not observed in previous SSRI trials. Adverse effects were consistent with current FDA listings. The authors were surprised that there was no difference between 20-mg and 40-mg dosages. A second large multicenter study of paroxetine (Tucker et al. 2001) found a mean dosage of 27 mg/day but also relatively equal proportions of patients at each dosage (10 mg–50 mg/day). This may suggest that flexible-dosage trials are increasing the dosage too quickly. However, it may also suggest that individual variability in dose–response is washed out in large comparisons. There are no dose comparisons for any other SSRI.

There are three additional published reports of placebo-controlled trials of an SSRI with positive findings, all with fluoxetine (Connor et al. 1999; Martenyi et al. 2002; Van der Kolk et al. 1994). A small placebo-controlled trial in U.S. veterans with fluoxetine reported negative results (Hertzberg et al. 2000).

Van der Kolk et al. (1994) reported a double-blind, placebo-controlled trial of 5 weeks of fluoxetine treatment in 31 subjects with combat-related PTSD and 33 patients with non-combat-related PTSD. Of the total sample, 54.8% also met criteria for major depression. Among those who completed the protocol (73.4% of the sample), fluoxetine (mean dosage, 40 mg/day at week 5) was found superior to placebo in reducing CAPS scores using analysis of covariance. Reduction of symptom severity (CAPS score) was approximately 40% for fluoxetine versus 15% for placebo in noncombat trauma victims. Fluoxetine was not superior to placebo in war veterans. Unfortunately, that report did not present intent-to-treat analyses, global response rates, symptom scores for the civilian subsample, or assessment of high end-state functioning. In the subgroup of civilians, fluoxetine was superior to placebo in reducing the numbing symptoms of Criterion C, but not avoidance, hyperarousal, or reexperiencing symptoms.

Connor et al. (1999) reported a 12-week placebo-controlled trial of fluoxetine in adult civilians with chronic PTSD (N=53; median years with PTSD, 6). A flexible dosage design was used (10 mg daily, increased to a maximum of 60 mg; median daily dosage in the last 3 weeks, 40 mg). Two-thirds of the subjects completed the full 12 weeks (36 of 53). Fluoxetine was rated superior to placebo, although both groups had high response rates (85% vs. 62%). Fluoxetine-treated patients were significantly more likely to be rated very much improved (59% vs. 19%). Forty-one percent (11 of 27) of fluoxetine-treated patients were rated as fully recovered, compared with 4% (1 of 26) of placebo-treated patients, suggesting that 60% of the sample remained symptomatic despite fluoxetine treatment.

In summary, the SSRIs are effective for chronic PTSD, reduce symptoms by about 50% acutely, and on average leave patients with a moderate degree of residual PTSD symptoms. We recommend continuing SSRI treatment for at least 1 year, since it appears that relapse risk is increased if treatment is discontinued at 6 months (Davidson et al. 2001a).

Tricyclic Compounds

Davidson et al. (1990) conducted an 8-week double-blind trial of amitriptyline (doses between 150 and 300 mg/day) in U.S. war veterans (N=62, dropout rate 26%). In the completer analysis only, the study found modest differences between drug and placebo on measures of anxiety and depression and overall severity, but not on PTSD symptoms. A second study of imipramine found somewhat more promising results (reviewed in the following section; Kosten et al. 1991). Modest results in these studies could be entirely due to the patient population studied (U.S. war veterans), however, and TCAs have not been studied in persons with PTSD attributable to other kinds of trauma.

Monoamine Oxidase Inhibitors

In the only study that compared two active treatments, Kosten et al. (1991) found both imipramine and phenelzine superior to placebo in an 8-week randomized controlled study of 60 war veterans with PTSD. This was a somewhat unusual sample in that no patients met criteria for major depression, although 47% met Research Diagnostic Criteria (RDC) for minor depression. Tricyclic blood levels and platelet monoamine oxidase inhibition were monitored in this study. The mean maximum dosage of imipramine was 225 mg/day, with a mean blood level of imipramine plus desipramine of 184±80 ng/mL at weeks 2–4. Mean maximum dosage of phenelzine was 68 mg/day, with a mean platelet monoamine oxidase activity of 94%±7%.

Retention in the study was 90% for the first 3 weeks, but only 31 of 60 subjects completed the full 8 weeks. Treatment retention was significantly better for phenelzine than for imipramine or placebo. An intent-to-treat analysis found that global improvement with imipramine (65%) and phenelzine (68%) was comparable, and superior to that with placebo (28%). However, on a continuous measure of PTSD symptoms (the Impact of Event Scale), phenelzine produced a significantly greater reduction in scores: 45%, as compared with a 25% drop for imipramine and a 5% drop for placebo.

Mood Stabilizers

There are many case reports and open trials of the range of available mood stabilizers for PTSD. These mood stabilizers include lithium, carbamazepine, valproic acid, and topiramate. Usually they are used as an adjunct to another medication that has been partially effective (e.g., an SSRI). Unfortunately there are few well-controlled trials, although a small controlled trial supports the efficacy of lamotrigine for PTSD (Hertzberg et al. 1999). A number of early uncontrolled studies reported success in patients with PTSD and prominent affective instability and/or explosive behavior.

Antiadrenergic Compounds

One of the earliest medication reports described the use of propranolol and clonidine to reduce hyperarousal symptoms in PTSD (Kolb et al. 1984). There are also no controlled trials with these compounds, but open trials and case reports have described their use as adjunctive treatments to reduce hyperarousal and, with clonidine and guanfacine in particular, to treat refractory nightmares in both children and adults.

Benzodiazepines

A small controlled trial found alprazolam to be only minimally effective among combat veterans and to have only nonspecific antianxiety effects. An open trial of clonazepam with a matched comparison group found more concerning results. Individuals treated with clonazepam were more likely to develop chronic PTSD than those who did not receive a benzodiazepine. Because of both these results and the fact that there are high rates of alcohol abuse in PTSD, clinicians should conduct careful assessments before prescribing these medications for insomnia. At best, they might be used in a time-limited fashion to reduce anxiety while slower-acting medications are being taken.

Newer Medications

Promising findings from open trials and case reports have been described for a number of compounds that have initially shown efficacy for depression, seizure disorders, or psychotic disorders, including fluvoxamine, trazodone, nefazodone, venlafaxine, mirtazapine, risperidone, and olanzapine. It is unclear whether these medications will prove superior to SSRIs, but anecdotal success in reducing symptoms without inducing sexual side effects has been described.

Psychotherapy

Early Psychodynamic History

Horowitz (1986) elaborated on Freud's theory that overwhelming experience can lead to psychopathology and developed a psychodynamic model based on faulty information processing. In Horowitz's model, the traumatized individual is overwhelmed with information, and either intrusive memories or numbing and denial of memory result as an attempt to process the information. Lindy et al. (1988) reported an open series of 37 Vietnam War veterans with PTSD who received psychodynamic psychotherapy aimed at processing traumatic war memories and compared them with a volunteer sample ($n=200$) of Vietnam veterans culled from clinical and nonclinical sources. After an average of 56 sessions, significant changes were noted by independent raters on the Hopkins Symptom Checklist-90, Impact of Events Scale, and the Cincinnati Stress Response Schedule. Intrusive phenomena, feelings of alienation and depression, and associated hostility and substance abuse were most notably changed. The confrontation of and management of intense rage in the victim is vital, according to many of these reports.

A comparative psychotherapy study randomly assigned patients with PTSD, as described by DSM-III, of no more than 5 years' duration ($N=112$)

to one of four groups: desensitization therapy, hypnotherapy, brief dynamic therapy, or wait-list control (Brom et al. 1989). Overall analyses found no significant differences between the three therapies, which were superior to the control condition. The number of dropouts was minimal ($n = 12$). Desensitization therapy reduced symptoms by 41.4%, compared with reductions of 33.7% for hypnotherapy and 29.4% for dynamic therapy. That is, desensitization therapy produced the largest acute reduction in PTSD symptoms, although differences were not statistically significant.

Cognitive-Behavioral Therapy for Acute Stress Disorder

A small nonrandomized trial in women with full PTSD symptoms within 30 days of trauma ($N=20$) compared a brief (four-session) cognitive-behavioral therapy (CBT) intervention based on established PTSD treatments to an assessment-only group (Foa et al. 1995). Two months after assault, the CBT group was significantly more improved, but this difference largely disappeared by about 6 months after assault.

The first randomized trial of ASD compared a similar brief (five-session) CBT intervention to supportive counseling (Bryant et al. 1998). At completion and 6-month follow-up reevaluation, the CBT group had reduced rates of PTSD compared with the counseling group. In a subsequent study ($N=45$) comparing two versions of CBT (exposure therapy plus cognitive therapy or exposure therapy alone) to supportive counseling, rates of PTSD 6 months later were approximately 20% in both CBT groups, compared with 67% in the control condition (Bryant et al. 1999).

Although all randomized trials to date have focused on people with ASD, it is probable that the same approach would be effective for those with acute PTSD symptoms but not prominent dissociative features.

Cognitive-Behavioral Therapy for Posttraumatic Stress Disorder

Several brief CBT programs have been found to be highly effective in ameliorating PTSD symptoms and related psychopathology. Arising from an experimental background, cognitive-behavioral interventions typically have been subjected to rigorous testing and traditionally involve repeated assessments of target symptoms, comparison groups, and well-delineated and replicable procedures. Because of the strength of the literature in this area, only well-controlled studies of CBT techniques for PTSD are reviewed here.

One set of cognitive-behavioral approaches employed with PTSD patients is exposure treatment, in which patients confront feared situations. This approach is designed to activate memories of the trauma to modify the pathological aspects of those memories (Foa and Rothbaum 1998). Obviously, the use of exposure techniques requires that the patient remember at least some details of the trauma. In another approach, anxiety management training (AMT), the focus is on management of fear by teaching patients skills for controlling their anxiety.

Prolonged Exposure

Exposure treatments for PTSD involve repeated reliving of the trauma with the aim of facilitating the processing of the trauma, which is thought to be impaired in survivors with chronic PTSD (Foa et al. 1989). Exposure treatment, as delivered by Foa and Rothbaum (1998), incorporates imaginal exposure (IE), in which the patient relives the trauma in his or her imagination and describes it out loud in the present tense in the therapy session. Other forms of exposure include in vivo exposure, in which patients confront realistically safe situations, places, or objects repeatedly that are reminders of the trauma until they no longer elicit such strong emotions. Some therapists have patients write repeatedly about the trauma as a form of exposure (e.g., Resick and Schnicke 1993). Early controlled studies of exposure therapy in PTSD were conducted with male Vietnam veterans. Exposure therapy was found to be modestly effective compared with standard treatment alone (weekly group/individual therapy) (Cooper and Clum 1989), compared with no treatment (Keane et al. 1989), and compared with traditional psychotherapy (Boudewyns et al. 1990).

Psychosocial treatment for PTSD related to other types of trauma has been considerably more promising. Rape victims with chronic PTSD were randomly assigned to nine sessions over 5 weeks of prolonged exposure (PE), stress inoculation training (SIT), supportive counseling (SC), or wait-list (WL) control (Foa et al. 1991). The SC treatment emphasized problem solving in the here and now and discouraged detailed discussion of the traumatic experience. A completer analysis was reported (N=45). Immediately after treatment, SIT was superior on a measure of PTSD severity to WL and SC. After treatment, 50% of patients receiving SIT, 40% of patients receiving PE,

90% of those receiving SC, and 100% of wait-listed patients still met criteria for PTSD. In the PE completer group, symptoms were reduced 59%, compared with a reduction of 46% for the SIT group and 22% for the SC group. It is of interest that in the SC and WL groups, arousal symptoms improved, but not intrusion and avoidance symptoms, suggesting that confronting the trauma in therapy is important to reduce intrusion and avoidance specifically.

A second randomized study compared the efficacy of nine twice-weekly sessions of PE, SIT, their combination (PE+SIT), and a WL comparison group in 96 female assault victims with PTSD (Foa et al. 1999). The authors had hypothesized that combination treatment might be more effective than either treatment alone. However, at completion of the trial, there were no differences between active treatments, and all were superior to WL. In the intent-to-treat sample, high end-state functioning (defined as test scores as follows: Post-traumatic Stress Symptom Scale—Interview Version [PSS-I], <20; State portion of State-Trait Anxiety Inventory [STAI-St], <40; Beck Depression Inventory [BDI], <10) was achieved by 52% in PE, 31% in SIT, 27% in PE+SIT, and 0% in WL. These differences achieved significance between PE and PE+SIT on chi-square analyses (P=0.05). The effect sizes (Cohen's d statistics) in the intent-to-treat sample on the PSS-I, the primary measure of PTSD symptoms, were the following: PE, 1.46; SIT, 0.85; PE+SIT, 0.82. Symptom reduction after treatment was 60% for PE, 56% for SIT, 55% for PE+SIT, and 18% for WL. At 1-year follow-up evaluation (N=46), all of the active treatments were equally effective on high end-state functioning (52%, PE; 42%, SIT; 36%, PE+SIT).

Other studies provide support for the efficacy of exposure treatment for PTSD in samples heterogeneous with regard to their traumas. Richards et al. (1994) treated 14 participants with PTSD with either four sessions of IE followed by four sessions of in vivo exposure, or in vivo followed by IE. Patients in both treatment conditions improved considerably, with no patients meeting criteria for PTSD at post-treatment evaluation or at 1-year follow-up evaluation. In a similar study in the United Kingdom, Marks et al. (1998) compared exposure therapy (EX), cognitive restructuring (CR), exposure therapy combined with cognitive restructuring (EX+CR), and relaxation training (RT) in adults with PTSD of at least 6 months' duration in a sample of patients with a history of mixed trauma. Data on those completing at least 6 weeks of treatment were analyzed (N=76). Immediately after treatment, results for the EX, CR, and EX+CR groups appeared to be superior to those for RT. When high end-state function was defined stringently as a 50% drop in PTSD symptoms, BDI<7, and STAI-St<5, response rates were 53% for EX, 32% for CR, 32% for EX+CR, and 15% for RT, not significantly different between groups. This study used CAPS scores, thus simplifying comparisons to our pilot data. The PE group scores were reduced from approximately 62 to 32, a 48% reduction. Symptom reductions in the other cells were 48% (CR), 51% (EX+CR), and 25% (RT).

Another UK study randomly assigned 72 patients to either IE or cognitive therapy (CT) after a 4-week evaluation and monitoring period (Tarrier et al. 1999). Type of trauma included crime (52%), accident (34%), and other (15%). Both treatments resulted in significant improvement compared to baseline, with no differences between treatments. CAPS score changes were from 71 to 48 for IE, a 32% reduction, and from 77 to 50 for CT, a 35% reduction. The percentage of patients rated as having none or slight symptoms after treatment did not differ between treatments: 41% for IE versus 33% for CT. The authors concluded there were no significant differences in the efficacy of IE versus that of CT. Another study that found eight weekly sessions of IE and in vivo exposure were effective in treating 23 participants with PTSD (Thompson et al. 1995).

The results from the studies discussed above offer support for the efficacy of imaginal and in vivo exposure for the treatment of PTSD resulting from a variety of traumas. In fact, no other intervention for PTSD has received more support than EX (Rothbaum et al. 2000).

Eye Movement Desensitization and Reprocessing

Eye movement desensitization and reprocessing (EMDR) (Shapiro 1995) involves the patient's imagining a traumatic scene and focusing on the accompanying cognitive and physical responses while the patient tracks the therapist's two fingers moving across the patient's visual field. This is repeated until discomfort decreases, at which point the patient is instructed to generate a more adaptive thought and to associate it with the scene while moving his or her eyes. In a critical review of the literature in the treatment guidelines generated by a task force for the International Society for Traumatic Stress Studies, EMDR was deemed to be an efficacious treatment for PTSD (Chemtob et al. 2000). The results of seven controlled published studies found large effect sizes for EMDR. The necessity of the eye movements has been called into question by some dismantling studies, but better-controlled studies are required to shed more light on the role of the eye movements.

There have been three controlled studies comparing EMDR to other treatments that included exposure. One published clinical trial compared eight sessions of EMDR to nine sessions of exposure-based therapy (Trauma Treatment Protocol [TTP]) for individuals with non-combat-related PTSD (N=32) (Devilly and Spence 1999). This relatively small study had a number of significant limitations, including the absence of randomized assignment and structured diagnostic interviews, nonstandardization of concurrent treatment (43% were also taking medication), small sample size, and analysis of only a completer sample. TTP also included elements of cognitive restructuring during and immediately after exposure. Findings must therefore be considered preliminary and limited with respect to comparison to PE. Both treatments produced significant improvement relative to baseline, and there were no significant differences between treatments on multiple analyses. Symptom reduction measured by the PSS-Symptom Reduction scale (Foa et al. 1993) was 60% for TTP and 29.8% for EMDR. At 3-month follow-up evaluation, treatment gains in the TTP group were stable, whereas the EMDR group showed a nonsignificant increase in symptoms. Using the method of Foa et al. (1991) to identify subjects with minimal symptoms at completion, the authors found that TTP was significantly superior to EMDR on four PTSD measures both immediately after treatment and at 3-month follow-up evaluation.

An unpublished controlled study aimed to evaluate the relative efficacy of PE and EMDR compared to a no-treatment WL control in the treatment of PTSD in 74 adult female rape victims. PE and EMDR were found to be equally effective immediately after treatment, but differences emerged at the 6-month follow-up evaluation favoring PE (Rothbaum et al. 2001). Another unpublished study (Taylor et al. 2001) compared EMDR to RT and EX. EX was found to be superior at posttreatment and follow-up evaluations, whereas EMDR and RT did not differ from one another in effectiveness.

Anxiety Management Training

AMT, another CBT approach shown to be helpful in treating PTSD, involves teaching patients skills to control their anxiety. The AMT program that has received the most attention is SIT, initially developed for survivors who remained highly fearful 3 months after being raped (Veronen and Kilpatrick 1983). SIT typically consists of education and training in coping skills, including deep muscle relaxation training, breathing control, role-playing, covert modeling, thought-stopping, and guided self-dialogue. The skills taught in SIT aim to decrease the anxiety experienced by rape survivors in many different situations. SIT was included in the studies by Foa et al. (1991, 1999) described above under "Prolonged Exposure." Overall, SIT produced decreases in PTSD and related symptoms at posttreatment and follow-up evaluations. These improvements were significantly greater than in the control conditions but not significantly greater than those produced by PE. SIT has also been found helpful when delivered in a group setting to rape survivors (Resick et al. 1988).

Other anxiety-management techniques, such as RT and CT, have also been studied in treating PTSD. A controlled study comparing three different forms of relaxation (relaxation, relaxation plus deep breathing, and relaxation plus deep breathing and biofeedback) for 90 Vietnam War veterans (Watson et al. 1997) found that all treatments were equally, but only mildly, effective in leading to improvement. CT and systematic desensitization both led to significant improvement in rape survivors (Frank and Stewart 1984; Frank et al. 1988). Self-exposure plus cognitive restructuring was superior, at posttreatment and follow-up evaluation, to progressive RT in 20 female sexual assault survivors (Echeburua et al. 1997).

One treatment that has been developed for rape survivors combines a number of techniques. Cognitive processing therapy (CPT) includes education, exposure by means of writing about the assault and sharing it in a group, and cognitive restructuring components. In a controlled trial for rape survivors comparing CPT, PE, and WL control groups, both treatment groups were significantly more improved than the control group and CPT and PE were equally effective in reducing PTSD (Resick et al. 2002).

Conclusion

Several manualized time-limited psychotherapies have been developed and validated in controlled trials, of which the best studied is prolonged exposure therapy. These treatments draw from a long tradition of trauma-focused psychotherapy and include in-depth assessments, psychoeducation, techniques that build the therapeutic alliance, systematic reconstruction of the traumatic experience in narrative form, and outside assignments designed to help the patient overcome often debilitating avoidance patterns.

Recent multicenter trials have shown SSRIs to be effective for chronic PTSD induced by a range of traumatic events. Trials in U.S. war veterans, however, have been less successful. This is likely due to the inclusion of patients with largely treatment-refractory PTSD in these trials, because anecdotal evidence and recent multinational trials with veterans from other combat situations have shown response rates comparable to those in U.S. civilian trials.

In the absence of additional controlled trials, results of a single modestly positive trial with U.S. war veterans indicate that tricyclic antidepressants may also be used. A single trial also showed good results with phenelzine, a monoamine oxidase inhibitor. A number of other compounds have shown promise in open trials and case reports, including mood stabilizers, antiadrenergic compounds, and atypical antipsychotics. These drugs are usually used in combination with validated medications to treat refractory symptom clusters such as insomnia, nightmares, and affective instability.

Surprisingly, there are no trials comparing psychotherapy to medication for adults with PTSD, and methodological differences between therapy and medication trials make comparisons largely uninterpretable. Moreover, there are no controlled trials examining combination treatments. A case series did, however, find that trauma-focused psychotherapy resulted in further improvement in a medication nonresponder and two partial responders to an SSRI, consistent with the view that these treatments have complementary, rather than redundant, mechanisms of action (Marshall et al. 2003).

In practice, many clinicians combine psychotherapy and medication, particularly for the most severely ill patients. At times, treatment with medication may facilitate participation in a trauma-focused psychotherapy, which requires motivation to overcome avoidance and a willingness to practice and master techniques designed to reduce anxiety and promote a shift toward greater mastery over and control of the traumatic memory.

References

American Psychiatric Association: Diagnostic and Statistical Manual of Mental Disorders, 3rd Edition. Washington, DC, American Psychiatric Association, 1980

American Psychiatric Association: Diagnostic and Statistical Manual of Mental Disorders, 3rd Edition, Revised. Washington, DC, American Psychiatric Association, 1987

American Psychiatric Association: Diagnostic and Statistical Manual of Mental Disorders, 4th Edition, Text Revision. Washington, DC, American Psychiatric Association, 2000

Australian Bureau of Statistics: Mental Health and Wellbeing: Profile of Adults. Canberra, Australia, Australian Bureau of Statistics, 1998

Beckham JC, Lytle BL, Feldman ME: Caregiver burden in partners of Vietnam war veterans with posttraumatic stress disorder. J Consult Clin Psychol 64:1068–1072, 1996

Blake DD, Weathers FW, Nagy LM, et al: The development of a clinician-administered PTSD scale. J Trauma Stress 8:75–90, 1995

Blanchard EB, Buckley TC, Hickling EJ, et al: Posttraumatic stress disorder and comorbid major depression: is the correlation an illusion? J Anxiety Disord 12:21–37, 1998

Boudewyns PA, Hyer L, Woods MG, et al: PTSD among Vietnam veterans: an early look at treatment outcome using direct therapeutic exposure. J Trauma Stress 3:359–368, 1990

Brady K, Pearlstein T, Asnis GM, et al: Efficacy and safety of sertraline treatment of posttraumatic stress disorder: a randomized controlled trial. JAMA 283:1837–1844, 2000

Brand AH, Johnson JH: Note on reliability of the Life Events Checklist. Psychol Rep 50:1274, 1982

Brom D, Kleber RJ, Defares PB: Brief psychotherapy for posttraumatic stress disorders. J Consult Clin Psychol 57:607–612, 1989

Bryant RA, Harvey AG, Dang ST, et al: Treatment of acute stress disorder: a comparison of cognitive-behavioral therapy and supportive counseling. J Consult Clin Psychol 66:862–866, 1998

Bryant RA, Sackville T, Dang ST, et al: Treating acute stress disorder: an evaluation of cognitive behavior therapy and counseling techniques. Am J Psychiatry 156:1780–1786, 1999

Chemtob CM, Tolin DF, Van Der Kolk BA, et al: Guidelines for treatment of PTSD: eye movement desensitization and reprocessing. J Trauma Stress 13:569–570, 2000

Cloitre M, Scarvalone P, Difede JA: Posttraumatic stress disorder, self- and interpersonal dysfunction among sexually retraumatized women. J Trauma Stress 10:473–482, 1997

Connor KM, Sutherland SM, Tupler LA, et al: Fluoxetine in post-traumatic stress disorder: randomized, double blind study. Br J Psychiatry 175:17–22, 1999

Cooper NA, Clum GA: Imaginal flooding as a supplementary treatment for PTSD in combat veterans: a controlled study. Behav Ther 3:381–391, 1989

Cordova MJ, Andrykowski MA, Kenady DE, et al: Frequency and correlates of post-traumatic-stress-disorder-like symptoms after treatment for breast cancer. J Consult Clin Psychol 63:981–986, 1995

Davidson J[R], Kudler H, Smith R, et al: Treatment of posttraumatic stress disorder with amitriptyline and placebo. Arch Gen Psychiatry 47:259–266, 1990

Davidson JR, Hughes D, Blazer DG, et al: Posttraumatic stress disorder in the community: an epidemiological study. Psychol Med 21:1–19, 1991

Davidson J[R], Pearlstein T, Londborg P, et al: Efficacy of sertraline in preventing relapse of posttraumatic stress disorder: results of a 28-week double-blind, placebo-controlled study. Am J Psychiatry 158:1974–1981, 2001a

Davidson JR, Rothbaum BO, van der Kolk B, et al: Multicenter, double-blind comparison of sertraline and placebo in the treatment of posttraumatic stress disorder. Arch Gen Psychiatry 58:485–492, 2001b

Delehanty DL, Raimonde AJ, Spoonster E: Initial posttraumatic urinary cortisol levels predict subsequent PTSD symptoms in motor vehicle accident victims. Biol Psychiatry 48:940–947, 2000

Devilly GJ, Spence SH: The relative efficacy and treatment distress of EMDR and a cognitive-behavioral treatment protocol in the amelioration of posttraumatic stress disorder. J Anxiety Disord 13:131–157, 1999

Echeburua E, de Corral P, Zubizarreta I, et al: Psychological treatment of chronic posttraumatic stress disorder in victims of sexual aggression. Behav Modif 21:433–456, 1997

Eilenberg J, Fullilove M, Goldman R, et al: Quality and use of trauma histories obtained from psychiatric outpatients through mandated inquiry. Psychiatr Serv 47:165–169, 1996

Foa EB, Rothbaum BO: Treating the Trauma of Rape: A Cognitive-Behavioral Therapy for PTSD. New York, Guilford, 1998

Foa EB, Steketee G, Rothbaum B: Behavioral/cognitive conceptualizations of posttraumatic stress disorder. Behav Ther 20:155–176, 1989

Foa EB, Rothbaum BO, Riggs DS, et al: Treatment of posttraumatic stress disorder in rape victims: a comparison between cognitive-behavioral procedures and counseling. J Consult Clin Psychol 59:715–723, 1991

Foa EB, Riggs DS, Dancu CV, et al: Reliability and validity of a brief instrument for assessing post-traumatic stress disorder. J Trauma Stress 6:459–473, 1993

Foa EB, Hearst-Ikeda D, Perry KJ: Evaluation of a brief cognitive-behavioral program for the prevention of chronic PTSD in recent assault victims. J Consult Clin Psychol 63:948–955, 1995

Foa EB, Dancu CV, Hembree, EA, et al: A comparison of exposure therapy, stress inoculation training, and their combination in reducing posttraumatic stress disorder in female assault victims. J Consult Clin Psychol 67:194–200, 1999

Frank E, Stewart BD: Depressive symptoms in rape victims. J Affect Disord 1:269–277, 1984

Frank E, Anderson B, Stewart BD, et al: Efficacy of cognitive behavior therapy and systematic desensitization in the treatment of rape trauma. Behav Ther 19:403–420, 1988

Gilbertson MW, Shenton ME, Ciszewski A, et al: Smaller hippocampus volume predicts pathologic vulnerability to psychological trauma. Nat Neurosci 5:1242–1247, 2002

Grossman R, Buchsbaum MS, Yehuda R: Neuroimaging studies in post-traumatic stress disorder. Psychiatr Clin North Am 25:317–340, 2002

Harvey AG, Bryant RA: Acute stress disorder: a synthesis and critique. Psychol Bull 128:886–902, 2002

Heim C, Ehlert U, Hellhammer DH: The potential role of hypocortisolism in the pathophysiology of stress-related bodily disorders. Psychoneuroendocrinology 25:1–35, 2000

Herman J: Trauma and Recovery. New York, Basic Books, 1992

Hertzberg MA, Butterfield MI, Feldman ME, et al: A preliminary study of lamotrigine for the treatment of posttraumatic stress disorder. Biol Psychiatry 45:1226–1229, 1999

Hertzberg MA, Feldman ME, Beckham JC, et al: Lack of efficacy for fluoxetine in PTSD: a placebo controlled trial in combat veterans. Ann Clin Psychiatry 12:101–105, 2000

Horowitz MJ: Stress Response Syndromes, 2nd Edition. Northvale, NJ, Jason Aronson, 1986

Hull AM: Neuroimaging findings in post-traumatic stress disorder: systematic review. Br J Psychiatry 181:102–110, 2002

Jacobson A, Koehler JE, Jones-Brown C: The failure of routine assessment to detect histories of assault experienced by psychiatric patients. Hosp Community Psychiatry 38:386–389, 1987

Johnson JH, McCutcheon S: Assessing life stress in older children and adolescents: preliminary findings with the Life Events Checklist, in Stress and Anxiety, Vol 7. Edited by Sarason IG, Spielberger CD. Washington, DC, Hemisphere, 1980, pp 111–125

Keane TM, Fairbank JA, Caddell JM, et al: Implosive (flooding) therapy reduces symptoms of PTSD in Vietnam combat veterans. Behav Ther 20:245–260, 1989

Kendler KS, Karkowski LM, Prescott CA: Causal relationship between stressful life events and the onset of major depression. Am J Psychiatry 156:837–841, 1999

Kessler RC, Sonnega A, Bromet E, et al: Posttraumatic stress disorder in the National Comorbidity Survey. Arch Gen Psychiatry 52:1048–1060, 1995

Kolb LC, Burris BC, Griffiths S: Propranolol and clonidine in the treatment of the chronic post-traumatic stress disorders of war, in Posttraumatic Stress Disorder: Psychological and Biological Sequelae. Edited by van der Kolk BA. Washington, DC, American Psychiatric Press, 1984, pp 98–105

Kosten TR, Frank JB, Dan E, et al: Pharmacotherapy for posttraumatic stress disorder using phenelzine or imipramine. J Nerv Ment Dis 179:366–370, 1991

Lindy JD, Green B, Grace M: Vietnam: A Casebook. New York, Brunner/Mazel, 1988

Londborg PD, Hegel MT, Goldstein S, et al: Sertraline treatment of posttraumatic stress disorder: results of 24 weeks of open-label continuation treatment. J Clin Psychiatry 62:325–331, 2001

Marks I, Lovell K, Noshirvani H, et al: Treatment of post-traumatic stress disorder by exposure and/or cognitive restructuring: a controlled study. Arch Gen Psychiatry 55:317–325, 1998

Marshall RD, Spitzer R, Liebowitz MR: A review and critique of the new DSM-IV diagnosis of acute stress disorder. Am J Psychiatry 156:1677–1685, 1999

Marshall RD, Beebe K, Oldham M, et al: Efficacy and safety of paroxetine treatment for chronic PTSD: a fixed-dose, placebo controlled study. Am J Psychiatry 158:1982–1988, 2001a

Marshall RD, Olfson M, Hellman F, et al: Comorbidity, impairment, and suicidality in subthreshold PTSD. Am J Psychiatry 158:1467–1473, 2001b

Marshall RD, Carcamo JH, Blanco C, et al: Trauma-focused psychotherapy after a partial response to medication in PTSD: pilot observations. Am J Psychother 57:374–383, 2003

Martenyi F, Brown EB, Zhang H, et al: Fluoxetine vs placebo in prevention of relapse in posttraumatic stress disorder. Br J Psychiatry 181:315–320, 2002

McFarlane C, Atchison M, Rafalowicz E, et al: Physical symptoms in posttraumatic stress disorder. J Psychosom Res 38:715–726, 1994

Physicians' Desk Reference. Montvale, NJ, Thomson PDR, 2001

Pitman RK, Sanders KM, Zusman RM, et al: Pilot study of secondary prevention of posttraumatic stress disorder with propranolol. Biological Psychiatry 51:189–192, 2002

Rauch SL, van der Kolk BA, Fisler RE, et al: A symptom provocation study of posttraumatic stress disorder using positron emission tomography and script-driven imagery. Arch Gen Psychiatry 53:380–387, 1996

Resick PA, Schnicke MK: Cognitive Processing Therapy for Rape Victims: A Treatment Manual. Newbury Park, CA, Sage Publications, 1993

Resick PA, Jordan CG, Girelli SA, et al: A comparative victim study of behavioral group therapy for sexual assault victims. Behav Ther 19:385–401, 1988

Resick PA, Nishith P, Weaver TL, et al: A comparison of cognitive-processing therapy with prolonged exposure and a waiting condition for the treatment of chronic posttraumatic stress disorder in female rape victims. J Consult Clin Psychol 70:867–879, 2002

Richards DA, Lovell K, Marks IM: Post-traumatic stress disorder: evaluation of a behavioral treatment program. J Trauma Stress 7:669–680, 1994

Riggs DS, Byrne CA, Weathers FW, et al: The quality of the intimate relationships of male Vietnam veterans; problems associated with posttraumatic stress disorder. J Trauma Stress 111:87–102, 1998

Rothbaum, BO, Meadows EA, Resick P, et al: Cognitive-behavioral treatment position paper summary for the ISTSS Treatment Guidelines Committee. J Trauma Stress 13:558–563, 2000

Rothbaum BO, Astin M, Marsteller F: Prolonged exposure vs EMDR for PTSD rape victims. Presented at the annual meeting of the International Society for Traumatic Stress Studies, New Orleans, LA, December 2001

Shalev AY, Freedman S, Peri T, et al: Prospective study of posttraumatic stress disorder and depression following trauma. Am J Psychiatry 15:630–637, 1998

Shapiro F: Eye Movement Desensitization and Reprocessing: Basic Principles, Protocols, and Procedures. New York, Guilford, 1995

Stein MB, Walker JR, Hazen AL, et al: Full and partial posttraumatic stress disorder: findings from a community survey. Am J Psychiatry 154:1114–1119, 1997

Tarrier N, Pilgrim H, Sommerfield C, et al: A randomised trial of cognitive therapy and imaginal exposure in the treatment of chronic posttraumatic stress disorder. J Consult Clin Psychol 67:13–18, 1999

Taylor S, Thordarson DS, Maxfield L: Comparative efficacy, speed, and adverse effects of three PTSD treatments: exposure therapy, EMDR, and relaxation training. Presented at the World Congress of Behavioral and Cognitive Therapies, Vancouver, BC, Canada, July 2001

Thompson JA, Charlton PFC, Kerry R, et al: An open trial of exposure therapy based on deconditioning for post-traumatic stress disorder. Br J Clin Psychol 34:407–416, 1995

Tucker P, Zaninelli R, Yehuda R, et al: Paroxetine in the treatment of chronic posttrau-
    matic stress disorder: results of a placebo-controlled, flexible dosage trial. J Clin
    Psychiatry 62:860–868, 2001

Vaiva G, Ducrocq F, Jezequel K, et al: Immediate treatment with propranolol decreases
    PTSD two months after trauma. Biol Psychiatry (in press)

Van Der Kolk BA, Dreyfuss D, Michaels M, et al: Fluoxetine in posttraumatic stress
    disorder. J Clin Psychiatry 55:517–522, 1994

Veronen LJ, Kilpatrick DG: Stress management for rape victims, in Stress Reduction
    and Prevention. Edited by Meichenbaum D, Jaremko ME. New York, Plenum
    Press, 1983, pp 341–374

Watson CG, Tuorila JR, Vickers KS, et al: The efficacies of three relaxation regimens
    in the treatment of PTSD in Vietnam war veterans. J Clin Psychol 53:917–923,
    1997

Wenninger K, Heiman JR: Relating body image to psychological and sexual functioning
    in child sexual abuse survivors. J Trauma Stress 11:543–623, 1998

Wolfe J, Kimerling R: Gender issues in the assessment of posttraumatic stress disorder,
    in Assessing Psychological Trauma and PTSD. Edited by Wilson J, Keane TM.
    New York, Guilford, 1997, pp 192–238

Yehuda R: Posttraumatic stress disorder. N Engl J Med 346:108–114, 2002

7

Generalized Anxiety Disorder

Jonathan D. Huppert, Ph.D.

Moira Rynn, M.D.

Phenomenology

Symptoms

Although "anxiety neurosis" has long been described, generalized anxiety disorder (GAD) per se is a relatively new diagnosis. In DSM-III (American Psychiatric Association 1980), GAD was in some ways a "wastebasket" diagnosis that applied only to those who suffered from anxiety symptoms but did not meet diagnostic criteria for any of the other anxiety disorders. However, in DSM-III-R (American Psychiatric Association 1987) and DSM-IV (American Psychiatric Association 1994), GAD was increasingly conceptualized as an important independent disorder.

In DSM-IV-TR (American Psychiatric Association 2000), the diagnosis of GAD (Table 7–1) includes two major aspects: 1) uncontrollable, unrealis-

The authors thank Karl Rickels, M.D., for his helpful comments on this manuscript.

Table 7–1.   DSM-IV-TR diagnostic criteria for generalized anxiety disorder

A. Excessive anxiety and worry (apprehensive expectation), occurring more days than not for at least 6 months, about a number of events or activities (such as work or school performance).
B. The person finds it difficult to control the worry.
C. The anxiety and worry are associated with three (or more) of the following six symptoms (with at least some symptoms present for more days than not for the past 6 months).   **Note:** Only one item is required in children.
    (1) restlessness or feeling keyed up or on edge
    (2) being easily fatigued
    (3) difficulty concentrating or mind going blank
    (4) irritability
    (5) muscle tension
    (6) sleep disturbance (difficulty falling or staying asleep, or restless unsatisfying sleep)
D. The focus of the anxiety and worry is not confined to features of an Axis I disorder, e.g., the anxiety or worry is not about having a panic attack (as in panic disorder), being embarrassed in public (as in social phobia), being contaminated (as in obsessive-compulsive disorder), being away from home or close relatives (as in separation anxiety disorder), gaining weight (as in anorexia nervosa), having multiple physical complaints (as in somatization disorder), or having a serious illness (as in hypochondriasis), and the anxiety and worry do not occur exclusively during posttraumatic stress disorder.
E. The anxiety, worry, or physical symptoms cause clinically significant distress or impairment in social, occupational, or other important areas of functioning.
F. The disturbance is not due to the direct physiological effects of a substance (e.g., a drug of abuse, a medication) or a general medical condition (e.g., hyperthyroidism) and does not occur exclusively during a mood disorder, a psychotic disorder, or a pervasive developmental disorder.

tic worry about more than one topic and 2) accompanying physiological symptoms including muscle tension, difficulty sleeping, fatigue, restlessness or feeling keyed up/on edge, irritability, and difficulty concentrating. These symptoms must be relatively persistent for a 6-month period and be distressing or interfere with functioning to meet criteria for GAD.

In addition, if anxiety symptoms are better accounted for by another disorder, the diagnosis of GAD is not made (see "Differential Diagnosis" section below). According to DSM-IV-TR, the diagnosis of GAD cannot be made when the disorder's symptoms occur solely during an episode of a mood disorder (i.e., major depression or dysthymia). The basic assumption behind this decision is that most individuals who are depressed are also anxious (Barlow 2002). Substance use disorders and general medical disorders should also be excluded.

Associated Features

GAD may be associated with significant comorbidity and morbidity. Early authors did not see GAD as an independent entity, partly because comorbidity is so common. Nevertheless, rates of comorbidity in GAD are no higher than those seen in depression. Furthermore, community studies demonstrate that the disability associated with GAD is as great as that associated with depression.

Whereas GAD typically starts in childhood or early adulthood, oftentimes a major stressor will exacerbate symptoms. Research (Wells 1994) and our clinical experience with GAD has led us to believe that people with GAD are often driven toward being perfectionistic, feel a greater need for control in their environment, have difficulty tolerating ambiguity, and feel increased personal responsibility for negative events that occur or are predicted to occur in their environment.

Epidemiology

GAD is a relatively common disorder. Judd et al. (1998), for example, reported a lifetime prevalence of SCID-diagnosed DSM-III-R GAD, using hierarchical exclusion rules for current panic and depression, of 3.6%. More recent results using DSM-III-R criteria, from the National Comorbidity Survey, found a 12-month prevalence of 3.1% and a lifetime prevalence of 5.1% (Wittchen et al. 1994). Furthermore, GAD is the most common anxiety disorder in primary care settings. GAD is approximately twice as common in females as in males.

A range of data indicate that GAD is a relatively chronic disorder (Brown et al. 1994). In view of such data, some argue that in contrast to other anxiety disorders, a subtype of GAD (chronic, pervasive symptoms since childhood) may be better conceptualized as an underlying personality trait that increases one's vulnerability to developing anxiety disorders per se (Sanderson and Wetzler 1991). However, recent research suggests that some anxiety disorders such as social phobia may be likely to precede GAD (Brown et al. 2001).

Table 7–2. General medical disorders associated with anxiety symptoms

Anemia
Arrhythmias
Angina
Asthma
Early dementia
Fibromyalgia
Gastroesophageal reflux disease
Hyperparathyroidism
Hyperthyroidism
Hypoglycemia
Irritable bowel syndrome
Mitral valve prolapse
Obstructive lung disease
Parkinson's disease
Paroxysmal atrial fibrillation
Pheochromocytoma
Pulmonary embolus
Substance abuse/withdrawal (including narcotics, benzodiazepines, and β-blockers)
Seizure disorders
Supraventricular tachycardia
Vestibular dysfunction

Assessment

Differential Diagnosis

Anxiety secondary to an underlying general medical disorder must be distinguished from GAD. Table 7–2 provides a list of general medical disorders that may be associated with anxiety symptoms.

Differentiating GAD from other anxiety disorders can be complicated. First, worry is a relatively generic feature of anxiety disorders (e.g., worry about panic attacks, worry about embarrassing oneself). In addition, there is a high level of comorbidity among the anxiety disorders and GAD in particular, which requires one to consider diagnosing multiple disorders as well as making differential diagnoses. The primary distinction between GAD and other anxiety disorders is the focus of the patient's concern. Patients with GAD experience uncontrollable worry about a number of different areas in their life. In fact, they often worry about their worrying (known as *metaworry;* Wells 1994). In contrast, the focus of concern for patients with other anxiety disorders is specific to their respective disorder.

Panic Disorder

Patients with panic disorder are worried about having a panic attack or the consequences of experiencing certain bodily sensations. Their focus is on internal states. What makes the differential diagnosis particularly confusing is that the worry experienced by patients with GAD can lead to a panic attack. However, unlike patients with panic disorder, patients with GAD are concerned primarily about some future event, not having a panic attack or the symptoms of anxiety per se. Another distinction is the course of onset of worry versus panic. Some patients with GAD are focused on the physical symptoms of their anxiety, and this can lead one to think that the preoccupation with bodily sensations is a sign of panic disorder. However, the onset of a panic attack is sudden and its peak typically lasts for several minutes, whereas the onset and course of GAD-related anxiety is usually longer and more stable.

Social Phobia

Because social concerns are a common area of worry for patients with GAD, they are often found to have comorbid social phobia (Sanderson et al. 1990). However, some guidelines for differentiating the two disorders can be made. The basic distinction is that GAD concerns are more global, focused on a number of different areas that may include social situations. In contrast, patients with social phobia are specifically concerned with being evaluated, embarrassed, or humiliated in front of others.

Obsessive-Compulsive Disorder

Although the differentiation between obsessive-compulsive disorder (OCD) and GAD seems obvious because of the behavioral rituals that are unique to OCD (Brown et al. 1994, 2001), there are still some cases that can be extremely difficult to differentiate. This is especially true of patients with OCD who do not have compulsions or have only mental rituals. The differentiation can be made, however, by assessing the focus of concern. Obsessions are focused on exaggerated or unrealistic expectations and are usually short-lived (e.g., "If I don't seal this envelope correctly, my kids will be injured on the way home from school"). In addition, obsessions often take an "if-then" form (e.g., "If I do/don't do/think something, then something bad will happen") or include vivid imagery (Wells 1994). Worry, on the other hand, is usually focused on future negative events that are not caused by the patient. According to nonanxious subjects, worry lasts longer, is more distracting, and usually consists of predominantly verbal thoughts as opposed to images (Wells and Morrison 1994). The thought content of a worry may be specified in a "what if" fashion, without a consequence being stated ("What if I get ill?"). Another difficult aspect of the differentiation of GAD and OCD is the fact that patients with GAD may engage in reassurance-seeking behaviors that can be somewhat ritualistic and superstitious. Patients with GAD may report feeling compelled to act to neutralize this worry (Wells and Morrison 1994) (e.g., to call one's wife at work to lessen a worry about something happening to her). However, these behaviors are not as consistent, methodical, or ritualized as compulsive behaviors in patients with OCD.

Mood Disorders

The final differentiation to be made is between GAD and mood disorders, especially major depression and dysthymia. More often than not, anxiety symptoms occur within the context of depression, and thus GAD is diagnosed as a separate disorder only when the symptoms have occurred at least at some point independent of depression. However, regardless of DSM exclusionary criteria, the nature of cognitions associated with each disorder can be distinguished: *ruminations* (common in depressive disorders) tend to be negative thought patterns about past events, whereas *worries* (associated with GAD) tend to be negative thought patterns about future events. This is consistent with theoretical conceptualizations of anxiety and depression that posit that depression is a reaction to uncontrollable, inescapable negative events, leading to feelings of hopelessness and helplessness and deactivation, whereas anxiety is a reaction to uncontrollable negative events that the person attempts or plans to escape from. (For a more detailed explanation, see Barlow et al. 1996.) Brown et al. (2001) presented data suggesting that without the rule-out criteria, 90% of patients with diagnosed dysthymia and 67% of patients with diagnosed major depression would be found to have concurrent GAD, but that with the rule-out criteria, only 5% had diagnosed GAD.

Assessment Measures

A number of self-report and interviewer rating scales can be used to assess and diagnose GAD. There has been considerable controversy about the reliability of the Hamilton Anxiety Rating Scale (Ham-A; Hamilton 1959), but Shear et al. (2001) have recently developed a coding system that greatly improves the interrater reliability of this measure. In addition, for diagnostic purposes, the Anxiety Disorders Interview Schedule for DSM-IV-TR has been shown to reliably diagnose GAD in terms of severity. (See Brown et al. 2001 for more details.) A number of self-report measures can be used to determine the severity of GAD. In our review of the literature, the only measure that was common to all outcome studies was the Beck Depression Inventory (Beck et al. 1961). However, there are other scales more specifically related to GAD, including the Penn State Worry Questionnaire (Meyer et al. 1990), which measures uncontrollable worry; the Depression, Anxiety, and Stress Scales (Lovibond and Lovibond 1995), which measures stress-related symptoms; and the GAD questionnaire for DSM-IV-TR (GADQ-IV; Newman et al. 2002), which follows DSM criteria for GAD. These have all been shown to differentiate GAD from other anxiety disorders.

Pathogenesis

Worry

Worry is the major cognitive component of GAD. People who have GAD tend to worry most of the day, nearly every day. However, worry in itself is not pathological. It is an attempt to predict future danger and/or an attempt to gain control over events that appear uncontrollable (and usually negative or dangerous). However, it is clear that pathological worry is dysfunctional in that it is, by definition, excessive and/or unrealistic and feels uncontrollable. As a result, patients overpredict the likelihood of negative events and exaggerate consequences if the events were to occur. In a study by Abel and Borkovec (1995), 100% of patients with GAD described their worry as uncontrollable, whereas none of the nonanxious control subjects did. In addition, anxious subjects tend to selectively attend to threatening, personally relevant stimuli (Mathews 1990). Frequently, there is an implied belief that worry will make the world more controllable and predictable. Consistent with this, worriers report five major functions of worry: 1) superstitious avoidance of catastrophes, 2) actual avoidance of catastrophes, 3) avoidance of deeper emotional topics, 4) coping preparation, and 5) motivating devices (Borkovec 1994).

Research supports the idea that pathological worry has a functional role for people with GAD. Ironically, worry inhibits autonomic arousal in patients with GAD when they are shown aversive imagery. Worrying may cause the avoidance of aversive imagery, which is associated with an even greater emotional arousal (Borkovec et al. 1991). Thus, worry may be maintained by both the avoidance of certain affective states and the reduction of anxious states through the decrease in arousal that occurs along with worry or by the latter alone. Research has recently supported the role of worry in avoidance of emotions (Mennin et al. 2003; Roemer and Orsillo 2002). Counterintuitively, relaxation has been shown to increase the amount of worry in some patients with GAD (Borkovec et al. 1991). It may be that for these patients relaxation signals a lack of control, triggering an increase in anxiety, or that patients sit quietly with their thoughts, causing greater exposure to their worries.

Somatic Symptoms

In addition to worry, patients with GAD experience unpleasant somatic sensations. Although these usually increase during the course of a worry episode, both the worry and the somatic sensations can be described as relatively persistent and pervasive. The most common somatic symptom reported by patients with GAD is muscle tension. Patients may experience other symptoms often associated with worry and tension, including irritability, restlessness, feeling keyed up or on edge, difficulty sleeping, fatigue, and difficulty concentrating.

Neurobiology

Multiple neurochemicals and neurotransmitter systems have been implicated as potential contributors to the development of GAD. These include the γ-aminobutyric acid (GABA)–benzodiazepine (BZ) complex, serotonin (5-HT), norepinephrine, cholecystokinin, corticotropin-releasing factor, the hypothalamic-pituitary-adrenal axis, and neurosteriods (Connor and Davidson 1998). Work on the GABA–BZ complex and the serotonin system is perhaps particularly relevant to the clinical setting and to current pharmacological treatments of GAD.

Indeed, in view of the link between early antianxiety treatments and GABA, it was logical to focus on the role of the GABA–BZ complex in GAD. Studies have shown a lower number of peripheral BZ binding sites on platelets and lymphocytes in patients with GAD. This finding was reversed when patients were treated with a BZ (Rocca et al. 1991; Weizman et al. 1987). The development of BZ ligands has allowed work demonstrating decreased BZ binding in the left temporal lobe.

A range of preclinical studies demonstrate that the 5-HT system plays an important role in mediating anxiety. Patients with GAD have a decrease of 5-HT in the cerebrospinal fluid (Brewerton et al. 1995) and reduced platelet paroxetine binding (Iny et al. 1994). Patients with GAD demonstrate exacerbation of anxiety symptoms after administration of the serotonin agonist *m*-chlorophenylpiperazine. In addition, several serotonergic agents are effective in the treatment of GAD.

Pharmacotherapy

The acute phase of anxiety in chronically anxious patients is managed best by anxiolytic medications such as BZs. However, remission of anxiety symptoms may not be sustained; less than 50% of chronically anxious patients will have sustained remission of symptoms after stopping acute medication treatment (Rickels and Schweizer 1990). Some chronically anxious patients may need to be treated for years. BZs have been used for a long time for the treatment of anxiety; however, they are sedating and with prolonged use do cause physical dependence (American Psychiatric Association 1990). Consequently, there has been a search for non-BZ anxiolytics; this initially produced buspirone and then the newer antidepressants (see Table 7–3).

Antidepressants

Given that comorbidity is common in GAD and that most antidepressants have shown treatment efficacy for GAD, antidepressants constitute a useful treatment choice for patients with GAD.

Tricyclic antidepressants such as imipramine have the advantages of single daily dosing and of well studied and readily available generic preparations, which may result in cost savings for some patients. The disadvantages are the delayed onset of a number of weeks, anticholinergic side effects, potentially associated weight gain, orthostatic hypotension side effects, and high overdose lethality. Imipramine is started at 25–50 mg/day and slowly increased each week. Therapeutic benefit is usually obtained at lower doses for GAD than for panic disorder, with the maximum dose of 300 mg. The main problem with this class of antidepressants is its side effect profile.

Table 7–3. Medications for generalized anxiety disorder

Class of medication	Dose range	Advantages	Disadvantages
Antidepressants			
Selective serotonin reuptake inhibitors	Fluoxetine, 20–60 mg Paroxetine, 20–60 mg Sertraline, 50–200 mg	Single daily dosing Effective at lower doses No concern with addiction Low lethality for overdose	Delay of onset of action Sexual dysfunction Weight gain Insomnia Discontinuation syndrome
Serotonin and noradrenaline reuptake inhibitor	Venlafaxine (extended release), 150–300 mg	Single daily dosing with an extended-release preparation No concern for addiction Low lethality for overdose	At higher doses, some incidence of increased blood pressure Nausea Insomnia Sexual dysfunction Withdrawal syndrome
Tricyclic antidepressants	Imipramine, 150–250 mg	Single daily dose Low cost of medication	Delayed onset of action High overdose lethality Anticholinergic Weight gain

Table 7–3. Medications for generalized anxiety disorder *(continued)*

Class of medication	Dose range	Advantages	Disadvantages
Benzodiazepines			
Long-acting	Diazepam, 5–15 mg Clonazepam, 0.5–2 mg	Long half-life Acute onset of action Withdrawal better tolerated Low cost of medication	Twice-daily dosing Sedation Withdrawal/dependence Affects motor coordination and memory Alcohol interaction
Short-acting	Alprazolam, 1–6 mg	Acute onset of action Low cost of medication	Short half-life Dosing three to four times a day Withdrawal/dependence Affects motor coordination and memory Alcohol interaction
Azaspirones			
Buspirone	15–60 mg	No concern with addiction Low lethality Treats comorbid major depressive disorder No motor or memory impairment No withdrawal or dependence	Twice-daily dosing May be less effective in patients also taking benzodiazepines Dizziness Nausea Headache

Venlafaxine, a serotonin-norepinephrine reuptake inhibitor (Rickels et al. 2000b), was the first antidepressant to receive U.S. Food and Drug Administration (FDA) approval for the treatment of GAD. Studies support both the short-term and long-term efficacy of this agent. Medication can be initiated at either 25 or 37.5mg/day, then titrated up to 75 mg/day of the sustained release form. The sustained-release form helps to minimize potential side effects. The onset of action is 2–4 weeks or longer. Side effects are nausea, sweating, dry mouth, blurred vision, dizziness, and sexual dysfunction. Some of these side effects, such as the nausea, diastolic hypertension, and sexual dysfunction, appear to be dose related.

Selective serotonin reuptake inhibitors (SSRIs) are increasingly used in the treatment of anxiety disorders. Recently, paroxetine has been approved by the FDA for the treatment of GAD (Pollack et al. 2001). The advantage of this group of antidepressants lies in their relative tolerability and safer side effect profile. Patients with GAD require usual antidepressant doses of the SSRIs, although in some cases it is useful to begin with a relatively low starting dose (e.g., sertraline, 25 mg/day; fluoxetine, 10 mg/day; paroxetine, 10 mg/day) before titrating upward. Side effects may include transient gastrointestinal effects, weight changes, and sexual dysfunction.

It appears that antidepressants work more slowly than BZs but are slightly more efficacious than buspirone after 8 weeks of treatment. Given the fact that many patients treated for GAD may require chronic or intermittent pharmacotherapy, it is important to choose an antidepressant that can be well tolerated over the long term.

Benzodiazepines

Multiple randomized double-blind trials, many of them placebo-controlled, have definitively demonstrated the efficacy of BZs in the acute treatment of GAD (Greenblatt and Shader 1983a, 1983b; Rickels and Schweizer 1990). BZs have an early onset of efficacy (1 week) and continue to demonstrate efficacy after 4–8 weeks. Studies have employed primarily diazepam and clorazepate or desmethyl diazepam but have also used alprazolam and lorazepam.

BZs are generally considered safe medications with a wide "therapeutic window" (Busto et al. 2000; Greenblatt and Shader 1983b; Rickels and Schweizer 1990). Nevertheless, a variety of behavioral adverse effects have been attributed to BZs, particularly when administered in higher doses. These include sedative, attentional, and memory-impaired effects; rebound anxiety; and physical dependence and discontinuation symptoms after prolonged use (Greenblatt and Shader 1983a; American Psychiatric Association 1990).

Tolerance to the sedative effects may develop early, despite continued anxiolytic effects. However, on withdrawal of BZs, particularly those with a short half-life, 20% or more of patients were found to temporarily have Ham-A scores that were equal or higher than their pretreatment baseline score, indicating a rebound anxiety that, it has been speculated, might be an early precursor of BZ withdrawal syndrome (Rickels et al. 1988). Other studies have reported similar rates of rebound anxiety when short-term BZ therapy was discontinued abruptly, ranging from 25% to 44% (Fontaine et al. 1984).

Alprazolam is often used for GAD, but its short half-life necessitates frequent dosing. The starting dose is 0.25–0.5 mg every 4–6 hours. The dose should be increased every 4–6 days until relief is obtained. Clonazepam is an alternative that has a longer half-life, which allows for less frequent dosing. It is started at a dose of 0.5 mg/day and increased to every 3–5 days until relief is obtained. Dependence may occur even after only a few weeks of use, and BZs must be discontinued carefully to avoid withdrawal symptoms.

Other than buspirone, BZs have until recently been the only class of drugs that was approved by the FDA for the treatment of GAD. Survey data (Balter and Uhlenhuth 1992) suggest that at least 10% of the adult population in the United States in 1990 had used a BZ at some time during the previous year. Recent community surveys found that almost 50% of patients meeting criteria for GAD have been treated with medication (Wittchen et al. 1994), with BZs being by far the most common class of drugs used (Woods et al. 1992). However, in view of their associated problems, BZs have been relegated by many physicians to treating only acute anxiety symptoms (Ashton 1994; Lader 1998).

Buspirone

Since the 1980s a number of double-blind studies, some of them placebo controlled, have confirmed buspirone's efficacy in the alleviation of anxiety symptoms in patients with GAD. Most of these were placebo lead-in, randomized, double-blind studies designed to minimize any placebo effect. The primary measure of efficacy was the Ham-A. One of the most salient clinical features of buspirone, compared with the BZs, is its gradual, relatively slow onset of action, with many patients' symptoms taking several weeks to respond. This slow onset makes buspirone less useful for the treatment of transient, situational, or acute anxiety and may account for the perception by some clinicians that buspirone is a slightly less effective anxiolytic than BZs (Deakin 1993).

A similar slow onset of action has been reported for the treatment of anxiety symptoms with antidepressants (Rickels et al. 1993). Psychic symptoms of anxiety such as worry, anger, irritability, and difficulty concentrating, which are diagnostically considered core features of GAD in DSM-IV-TR, respond better to buspirone when compared to BZs, whereas the reverse is true for somatic symptoms such as muscle tension and insomnia (Pecknold et al. 1989; Rickels et al. 1982). Similar observations have been made for antidepressant treatment of GAD (Rickels et al. 1993, 2000a).

5-HT_{1A} drugs such as buspirone appear to act as partial agonists at the postsynaptic 5-HT_{1A} population of serotonin receptors located in the hippocampus, but as full agonists at the presynaptic 5-HT_{1A} serotonergic autoreceptors located in the dorsal raphe nucleus. Binding to these receptors enables these drugs to influence the activity of serotonergic neurons through receptor down-regulation. Chronic administration of azapirones, as with traditional antidepressants, causes a down-regulation of 5-HT_2 receptors, possibly explaining their limited antidepressant properties. Thus, patients with GAD and subsyndromal depressive symptoms may also demonstrate a decrease in depressive symptoms during treatment with buspirone (Feighner et al. 1982).

Buspirone is 100% absorbed after oral administration (Jajoo et al. 1989). The oral bioavailability is approximately 5% after extensive first-pass metabolism, and a linear relationship between acute oral dose and area under the plasma concentration–time curve was demonstrated. The first-pass metabolism of buspirone is decreased by taking food with buspirone, but the clinical significance of these findings is not known. Buspirone is more than 95% bound to plasma proteins. It undergoes extensive metabolism so that less than 1% of an administered dose is excreted unchanged in the urine. There are seven major and five minor metabolites that have been identified; the major metabolic pathways are hydroxylation and dealkylation. The elimination half-life of buspirone in healthy subjects ranges from 2 to 11 hours.

Because buspirone does not exhibit cross-tolerance to BZs and thus does not block BZ withdrawal symptoms, patients should never be abruptly switched from a BZ to buspirone. When switching BZ-treated patients to buspirone, it is beneficial to initiate buspirone therapy concurrently for 2–4 weeks before tapering BZ gradually. Some studies in which BZ was abruptly replaced with buspirone have shown no benefit for buspirone facilitating BZ withdrawal, whereas other studies have shown some beneficial results when buspirone was started several weeks before the BZ taper process was initiated.

The recommended initial dosage of buspirone is 15 mg/day administered in 2–3 divided doses. The dosage should be increased to 30 mg daily to achieve an optimal therapeutic response. The recommended maximum daily dosage is 45 mg in the United Kingdom and 60 mg in the United States. There are no firm recommendations regarding dosage adjustments in patients with hepatic or renal insufficiency. Although there appears to be some reduction in the elimination of buspirone or the weakly active 1-(2-pyrimidinyl)–piperazine (1-PP) metabolite in such patients, interpatient variation in pharmacokinetic parameters is substantial. Nevertheless, dosage adjustments may be necessary in patients with severe renal or hepatic impairment. No age-related dosage adjustments are necessary in elderly patients.

The side effect profile of buspirone makes it a positive option for patients who do not require immediate relief of symptoms and who have not had previous treatment with a BZ. The most commonly reported adverse events are dizziness, nausea, headache, fatigue, lightheadedness, and dry mouth. There are very few published data on buspirone overdose, and the data that are available suggest that buspirone is not toxic in overdose. No deaths have been associated with an overdose of buspirone alone (Newton et al. 1986).

Hydroxyzine

Hydroxyzine is the only antihistamine that was studied in the early 1960s as an anxiolytic, and in the United States this agent has an indication for use in the symptomatic relief of "anxiety and tension associated with psychoneurosis" (Physicians' Desk Reference 2003). Hydroxyzine acts as an antagonist at H_1 receptors and to a lesser extent at muscarinic receptors and 5-HT_2 receptors. It has even less binding to α_1 and dopamine 2 receptors (Kubo et al. 1987; Snyder and Snowman 1987). A large multisite family practice study, for example, compared a low dose of hydroxyzine (50 mg/day), given in divided doses, to placebo (Darcis et al. 1995). Statistically significant differences in favor of hydroxyzine were present at week 4, and this improvement was maintained for 1 additional week while patients received a placebo. Thus, no evidence for discontinuation symptoms or withdrawal symptoms was observed after 4 weeks of hydroxyzine treatment. This provides an alternative for patients needing anxiolytic treatment who may not want or be appropriate candidates for BZ treatment even for the short term.

Maintenance Pharmacotherapy

There are limited empirical data to direct the length of GAD treatment. Rickels et al. (1991) found that 25% of patients who had been treated for an average of 8 years and had been without BZ treatment for 3 years still had marked levels of anxiety. It appears that GAD is a chronic problem. For most patients, it is perhaps advisable to continue therapy for 6–12 months and then to discuss with the patient a trial period without the medication, monitoring closely for signs of relapse. Patients with more persistent GAD may require long-term treatment.

Psychotherapy

In *Textbook of Anxiety Disorders*, we reported on all outcome studies that had been published since 1990 and briefly described a number of reviews (Huppert and Sanderson 2002). Here we summarize these findings. The Task Force of the Division of Clinical Psychology of the American Psychological Association, involved with identifying empirically supported treatments, has found that only techniques used in cognitive-behavioral therapy (CBT) meet criteria to be included as empirically supported treatments for GAD (Chambless et al. 1998; Woody and Sanderson 1998). Although preliminary evidence (Durham et al. 1994) suggests that both long- and short-term psychodynamic treatments for anxiety disorders may be effective, adequate controlled studies have yet to be conducted.

There have been eight studies conducted since the publication of DSM-III-R that have used these more conservative diagnostic criteria to examine the efficacy of CBT. Most studies have used CBT and at least one other treatment group, a minimum of a 6-month follow-up assessment, and a variety of outcome measures, usually a combination of clinician-rated and self-report measures. Possibly because of the fact that the eight studies used a variety of different methodologies and outcomes measures, there is a relatively wide range of improvement found across the studies. Consistently, improvement was rated greater by clinicians blinded to patients' treatment protocols than by patients' self-reports. Clinicians rated patients who participated in CBT to be improved between 34% and 68%; self-report measures yielded between 16% and 71% improvement. In addition, four of six studies showed further improvement at follow-up evaluation, whereas two showed no change. Behavior therapy or relaxation yielded slightly lower effects, with clinician ratings ranging between 17% and 61% and self-report measures showing between 11.3% and 42% change. Two studies showed continued improvement, two demonstrated maintained gains, and one reported deterioration at follow-up evaluation. The only other group reported in a number of studies was patients on a wait list, which demonstrated either no change or deterioration at both posttreatment and follow-up evaluations.

Most reviews have concluded that the effects of CBT, although significant and similar to most medications, are clinically modest and that improvements in treatment were still warranted. According to one review, studies that demonstrated the greatest effects were those that included patients who were not taking any medications. In addition, patients appeared to make greater treatment gains if they were recruited outside of psychiatric settings (e.g., by primary care physicians or through newspaper ads; Durham and Allan 1993). The data on the effect of comorbidity (both Axis I and Axis II) on outcome have been inconsistent (Durham and Allen 1993); however, presence of comorbid personality disorders likely increases dropout rates.

A number of techniques included among the treatments in the above-mentioned studies appear to have positive additive influence on treatment outcomes (Huppert and Sanderson 2002): psychoeducation, self-monitoring, cognitive restructuring, relaxation, worry exposure, and worry behavior control. These techniques should be taught in the context of a good therapeutic alliance. Each is discussed briefly below.

Psychoeducation

Providing education about GAD is a way to introduce the treatment rationale and thus possibly facilitate treatment compliance. We recommend that psychoeducation be first provided in written form and then discussed in a session.

Self-Monitoring

Self-monitoring is one of the most basic yet essential parts of CBT. Monitoring is used both as an assessment procedure (to identify the context and content of worry) and a treatment strategy (becoming aware of patterns and focusing on worry and anxiety may lead to reduction in anxiety and worry). Each time the patient feels anxious, he or she should record when, where, and the intensity of the experience, including what symptoms are present. The basic aspects of worry monitoring are date, time begun, time ended, place, event (trigger), average anxiety (on a scale from 1 to 8), peak anxiety (1–8), average depression (1–8), and topics of worry. Once cognitive restructuring is introduced, monitoring the specific thought process involving worries is added.

Cognitive Therapy: Restructuring the Worry

As stated above, worry is a predominantly cognitive process, thereby making cognition an important aspect of to be addressed. Cognitive therapy is an effective strategy for this purpose. Patients with anxiety disorders, and with GAD in particular, overestimate the likelihood of negative events and underestimate their ability to cope with difficult situations (Beck and Emery 1985). These cognitive distortions can play a major role in the vicious circle of anxiety, and they accentuate the patient's feelings of danger and threat. Thus, cognitive therapy targets the faulty appraisal system and attempts to guide the patient toward more realistic, logical thinking.

Relaxation

Relaxation exercises are an important component of most CBT-oriented treatments for GAD. Their function is to reduce the physiological correlates of worry and anxiety by lowering the patient's overall arousal level. Most recent methods of relaxation have adapted a flexible concept of teaching relaxation, rather than insisting on any particular method. Thus, although progressive muscle relaxation techniques are emphasized for most patients and have the most empirical support, if a patient prefers another method and is able to use it effectively, then we recommend continued use of that strategy.

Worry Exposure/Stimulus Control

Another technique that has been recently developed but has not gained empirical support to date is worry exposure. As noted above, perpetuation of worry in patients with GAD may be due to ineffective processing that is a result of avoiding concentration on the worry itself. Instead of focusing on a worry, patients attempt to avoid fully processing the worry through various behaviors, as well as through constant shifting of worries. Thus, Brown et al. (1993) described a technique in which patients purposely expose themselves to both worry and images associated with the worry for an extended period of time. The purpose is to have the patient activate the worst possible outcome in order to process it and habituate to the anxiety associated with it. Borkovec (1983) developed a similar technique that he referred to as "stimulus control."

Worry Behavior Prevention

Many patients who worry may behave in certain ways to try to avoid it. As noted, uncontrollable worry, although an aversive experience, may still serve the function of avoiding an even more intolerable experience (i.e., by focusing on the worry instead of the other experience). To prevent worry behaviors, the patient carefully monitors his or her actions when he or she notices the onset of worry. Both subtle and explicit variants of these avoidance behaviors are detected through careful monitoring, assessment, and questioning. Then, similar to what is done in the technique of response prevention used in the treatment of OCD, the patient is asked to refrain from these behaviors and instead to use the techniques described above to cope with the worry. If there are many behaviors or if the patient is too anxious to just give up the worry behaviors, hierarchies are created to assist the patient in systematically giving up the behaviors, starting with easier ones and moving on to more difficult behaviors, making the task considerably less overwhelming (e.g., checking the child's forehead once daily, then every other day, and so on).

Other Techniques

If some people with GAD are avoiding affect, then simply eliminating the worry through relaxation and cognitive techniques will not work unless they are taught other strategies to deal with the triggers for the affect. A number of groups are attempting to address these issues through different techniques. Borkovec (1997) proposed that interpersonal strategies (Safran and Segal 1990) and emotion-focused strategies (Greenberg and Safran 1987) be tested in addition to cognitive techniques, to see whether processing of interpersonal difficulties facilitates activation and modification of affective structures (Foa and Kozak 1986). Similarly, Mennin et al. (in press) are working on new cognitive-behavioral strategies to accomplish the same goals. Roemer et al. (2002) have worked on integrating treatment strategies from a form of therapy that focuses on preventing experiential and behavioral avoidance, called Acceptance and Commitment Therapy (Hayes et al. 1999). Sanderson and colleagues have used schema-focused therapy with those patients whose disorder had not responded to traditional CBT (McGinn et al. 1994). This approach focuses on addressing underlying "early maladaptive schemas" that theoretically influence current symptomatology. On the basis of these ideas, one of us (J.D.H.) has recently begun to use new strategies, including having the patient develop a list of all emotions, rank-ordering the difficulty he or she has in coping with them, and then going through a cognitive-behavioral analysis of each emotion (Huppert and Alley, in press). This is followed by a hierarchy of imaginal and in vivo situations that encourage the emotional experiences that have previously been avoided. Clinical experience suggests that these additional techniques may lead to further symptom improvement for patients with GAD.

Conclusion

GAD is a common, persistent, debilitating disorder that often goes untreated. Both pharmacological and psychosocial treatments, especially CBT, help alleviate many of the symptoms of GAD. However, more research is needed on how to further improve patients' quality of life and on the optimal combination and sequencing of CBT and medication.

References

Abel JL, Borkovec TD: Generalizability of DSM-III-R generalized anxiety disorders to proposed DSM-IV-TR criteria and cross validation of proposed changes. J Anxiety Disord 9:303–315, 1995

American Psychiatric Association: Benzodiazepine Dependence, Toxicity, and Abuse: A Task Force Report of the American Psychiatric Association. Washington, DC, American Psychiatric Association, 1990

American Psychiatric Association: Diagnostic and Statistical Manual of Mental Disorders, 3rd Edition. Washington, DC, American Psychiatric Association, 1980

American Psychiatric Association: Diagnostic and Statistical Manual of Mental Disorders, 3rd Edition, Revised. Washington, DC, American Psychiatric Association, 1987

American Psychiatric Association: Diagnostic and Statistical Manual of Mental Disorders, 4th Edition. Washington, DC, American Psychiatric Association, 1994

American Psychiatric Association: Diagnostic and Statistical Manual of Mental Disorders, 4th Edition, Text Revision. Washington, DC, American Psychiatric Association, 2000

Ashton H: Guidelines for the rational use of benzodiazepines: when and what to use. Drugs 48:25–40, 1994

Balter MB, Uhlenhuth EH: Prescribing and use of benzodiazepines: an epidemiologic perspective. J Psychoactive Drugs 24:63–64, 1992

Barlow DH: Anxiety and Its Disorders: The Nature and Treatment of Anxiety and Panic, 2nd Edition. New York, Guilford, 2002

Barlow DH, Chorpita BF, Turovsky J: Fear, panic, anxiety, and disorders of emotion, in Nebraska Symposium on Motivation: Perspectives on Anxiety, Panic, and Fear. Edited by Hope DA. Lincoln, NE, University of Nebraska Press, 1996, pp 251–328

Beck AT, Emery G: Anxiety Disorders and Phobias: A Cognitive Perspective. New York, Basic Books, 1985

Beck AT, Ward CH, Mendelson M, et al: An inventory for measuring depression. Arch Gen Psychiatry 41:561–571, 1961

Borkovec TD: The nature, functions, and origins of worry, in Worrying: Perspectives on Theory, Assessment and Treatment. Edited by Davey GCL, Tallis F. New York, Wiley, 1994, pp 5–33

Borkovec TD: Limitations of CBT for generalized anxiety disorder. Paper presented at the annual meeting of the British Association for Behavioural and Cognitive Therapy, Canterbury, England, July 1997

Borkovec TD, Wilkinson L, Folensbee R, et al: Stimulus control applications to the treatment of worry. Behav Res Ther 21:153–158, 1983

Borkovec TD, Shadick RN, Hopkins M: The nature of normal and pathological worry, in Chronic Anxiety, Generalized Anxiety Disorder, and Mixed Anxiety Depression. Edited by Rapee RM, Barlow DH. New York, Guilford, 1991, pp 29–51

Brewerton TD, Lydiard RB, Johnson M, et al: CSF serotonin: diagnostic and seasonal differences. Biol Psychiatry 37:655, 1995

Brown TA, O'Leary TA, Barlow DH: Generalized anxiety disorder, in Clinical Handbook of Psychological Disorders, 2nd Edition. Edited by Barlow DH. New York, Guilford, 1993, pp 137–188

Brown TA, Barlow DH, Liebowitz MR: The empirical basis of generalized anxiety disorder. Am J Psychiatry 151:1272–1280, 1994

Brown TA, Campbell LA, Lehman CL, et al: Current and lifetime comorbidity of the DSM-IV-TR anxiety and mood disorders in a large clinical sample. J Abnorm Psychol 110:585–599, 2001

Busto UE, Bremner KE, Knight K, et al: Long-term benzodiazepine therapy does not result in brain abnormalities. J Clin Psychiatry 20:2–6, 2000

Chambless DL, Gillis MM: Cognitive therapy of anxiety disorder. J Consult Clin Psychol 61:248–260, 1993

Chambless DL, Baker MJ, Baucom DH, et al: Update on empirically validated therapies, II. The Clinical Psychologist 51:3–16, 1998

Connor KM, Davidson JRT: Generalized anxiety disorder: neurobiological and pharmacotherapeutic perspectives. Biol Psychiatry 44:1286–1294, 1998

Darcis T, Ferreri M, Natens J, et al, the French GP Study Group for Hydroxyzine: A multicentre double-blind, placebo-controlled study investigating the anxiolytic efficacy of hydroxyzine in patients with generalized anxiety. Hum Psychopharmacol 10:181–187, 1995

Deakin JFW: A review of the clinical efficacy of 5-HT$_{1A}$ agonists in anxiety and depression. J Psychopharmacol 7:283–289, 1993

Durham RC, Allan T: Psychological treatment of generalized anxiety disorder: review of the clinical significance of results in outcome studies since 1980. Br J Psychiatry 163:19–26, 1993

Durham RC, Murphy T, Allan T, et al: Cognitive therapy, analytic psychotherapy and anxiety management training for generalized anxiety disorder. Br J Psychiatry 165:315–323, 1994

Feighner JP, Merideth CH, Hendrickson GA: A double-blind comparison of buspirone and diazepam in outpatients with generalized anxiety disorder. J Clin Psychiatry 43:103–107, 1982

Foa EB, Kozak MJ: Emotional processing of fear: exposure to corrective information. Psychol Bull 99:20–35, 1986

Fontaine R, Chouinard G, Annable L: Rebound anxiety in anxious patients after abrupt withdrawal of benzodiazepine treatment. Am J Psychiatry 141:848–852, 1984

Greenberg LS, Safran JD: Emotion in Psychotherapy: Affect, Cognition, and the Process of Change. New York, Guilford, 1987

Greenblatt DJ, Shader RI, Abernethy DR: Current status of benzodiazepines: part I. N Engl J Med 309:354–358,1983a

Greenblatt DJ, Shader RI, Abernethy DR: Current status of benzodiazepines: part II. N Engl J Med 309:410–416, 1983b

Hamilton MA: The assessment of anxiety states by rating. Br J Med Psychol 32:50–55, 1959

Hayes SC, Strosahl KD, Wilson KG: Acceptance and Commitment Therapy: An Experiential Approach to Behavior Change. New York, Guilford, 1999

Huppert JD, Alley AC: The clinical application of emotion research in generalized anxiety disorder: some proposed procedures. Cognitive and Behavioral Practice (in press)

Huppert JD, Sanderson WC: Psychotherapy for generalized anxiety disorder, in Textbook of Anxiety Disorders. Edited by Stein DJ, Hollander E. Washington, DC, American Psychiatric Publishing, 2002, pp 141–155

Iny LJ, Pecknold J, Suranyi-Cadotte BE, et al: Studies of a neurochemical link between depression, anxiety, and stress from [3H] imipramine and [3H] paroxetine binding on human platelets. Biol Psychiatry 36:281–291, 1994

Jajoo HK, Mayol RF, LaBudde JA, et al: Metabolism of the antianxiety drug buspirone in human subjects. Drug Metab Dispos 17:634–640, 1989

Judd LL, Kessler RC, Paulus MP, et al: Comorbidity as a fundamental feature of generalized anxiety disorders: results from the National Comorbidity Study (NCS). Acta Psychiatr Scand Suppl 393:6–11, 1998

Kubo N, Shirakawa T, Kuno T, et al: Antimuscarinic effects of antihistamines: quantitative evaluation by receptor-binding assay. Jpn J Pharmacol 43:277–281, 1987

Lader MH: The nature and duration of treatment for GAD. Acta Psychiatr Scand Suppl 393:109–117, 1998

Lovibond SH, Lovibond PF: Manual for the Depression Anxiety Stress Scales. Sydney, Australia, Psychology Foundation of Australia, 1995

Mathews A: Why worry? The cognitive function of anxiety. Behav Res Ther 28:455–468, 1990

McGinn LK, Young JE, Sanderson WC: When and how to do long-term therapy without feeling guilty. Cognitive and Behavioral Practice 2:187–212, 1994

Mennin DS, Turk CL, Heimberg RG, et al: Focusing on the regulation of emotion: a new direction for conceptualizing and treating generalized anxiety disorder, in Cognitive Therapy Over the Lifespan: Theory, Research and Practice. Edited by Reinecke MA, Clark DA. New York, Wiley, 2003

Meyer TJ, Miller ML, Metzger RL, et al: Development and validation of the Penn State Worry Questionnaire. Behav Res Ther 28:487–495, 1990

Newman MG, Zuellig AR, Kachin KE, et al: Preliminary reliability and validity of the Generalized Anxiety Disorder Questionnaire-IV: a revised self-report diagnostic measure of generalized anxiety disorder. Behav Ther 33:215–233, 2002

Newton RE, Marunycz JD, Alderdice MT, et al: Review of the side-effect profile of buspirone. Am J Med 80 (suppl 3B):17–21, 1986

Pecknold JC, Matas M, Howarth BG, et al: Evaluation of buspirone as an antianxiety agent: buspirone and diazepam vs placebo. Am J Psychiatry 34:766–771, 1989

Physicians' Desk Reference. Montvale, NJ, Thomson PDR, 2003

Pollack MH, Zaninelli R, Goddard A, et al: Paroxetine in the treatment of generalized anxiety disorder: results of a placebo-controlled, flexible-dosage trial. J Clin Psychiatry 62:350–357, 2001

Rickels K, Schweizer E: The clinical course and long-term management of generalized anxiety disorder: J Clin Psychopharmacol 10 (3 suppl):101S–110S, 1990

Rickels K, Wiseman K, Norstad N, et al: Buspirone and diazepam in anxiety: a controlled study. J Clin Psychiatry 43 (sec 2):81–86, 1982

Rickels K, Fox IL, Greenblatt DJ, et al: Clorazepate and lorazepam: clinical improvement and rebound anxiety. Am J Psychiatry 145:312–317, 1988

Rickels K, Case WG, Schweizer E, et al: Long-term benzodiazepine users: 3 years after participation in a discontinuation program. Am J Psychiatry 148:757–761, 1991

Rickels K, Downing R, Schweizer E, et al: Antidepressants for the treatment of generalized anxiety disorder: a placebo-controlled comparison of imipramine, trazodone, and diazepam. Arch Gen Psychiatry 50:884–895, 1993

Rickels K, DeMartinis N, Garcia-Espana F, et al: Imipramine and buspirone in treatment of patients with generalized anxiety disorder who are discontinuing long-term benzodiazepine therapy. Am J Psychiatry 157:1973–1979, 2000a

Rickels K, Pollack MH, Sheehan DV, et al: Efficacy of venlafaxine extended-release capsules in nondepressed outpatients with generalized anxiety disorder. Am J Psychiatry 157:968–974, 2000b

Rocca P, Ferrero P, Gualerzi, et al: Peripheral-type benzodiazepine receptors in anxiety disorders. Acta Psychiatr Scand 84:537–544, 1991

Roemer L, Orsillo SM: Expanding our conceptualization of and treatment for generalized anxiety disorder: integrating mindfulness/acceptance-based approaches with existing cognitive-behavioral models. Clin Psychol 9:54–68, 2002

Roemer L, Orsillo SM, Barlow DH: Generalized anxiety disorder, in Anxiety and Its Disorders: The Nature and Treatment of Anxiety and Panic, 2nd Edition. Edited by Barlow DH. New York, Guilford, 2002, pp 477–515

Sanderson WC, Wetzler S: Chronic anxiety and generalized anxiety disorder: issues in comorbidity, in Chronic Anxiety, Generalized Anxiety Disorder, and Mixed Anxiety Depression. Edited by Rapee R, Barlow DH. New York, Guilford, 1991, pp 119–135

Sanderson WC, DiNardo PA, Rapee RM, et al: Syndrome comorbidity in patients diagnosed with a DSM-III-R anxiety disorder. J Abnorm Psychol 99:308–312, 1990

Safran JD, Segal ZV: Interpersonal Process in Cognitive Therapy. New York, Basic Books, 1990

Shear MK, Vander Bilt J, Rucci P, et al: Reliability and validity of a structured guide for the Hamilton Anxiety Rating Scale (SIGH-A). Depress Anxiety 13:166–178, 2001

Snyder SH, Snowman AM: Receptor effects of cetirizine. Ann Allergy 59:4–8, 1987

Weizman R, Tanne Z, Granek M, et al: Peripheral benzodiazepine binding sites on platelet membranes are increased during diazepam treatment of anxious patients. Eur J Pharmacol 138:289–292, 1987

Wells A: Attention and the control of worry, in Worrying: Perspectives on Theory, Assessment and Treatment. Edited by Davey GCL, Tallis F. New York, Wiley, 1994, pp 91–114

Wells A, Morrison AP: Qualitative dimensions of normal worry and normal obsessions: a comparative study. Behav Res Ther 32:867–870, 1994

Wittchen H-U, Zhao S, Kessler RC, et al: DSM-III-R generalized anxiety disorder in the National Comorbidity Survey. Arch Gen Psychiatry 51:355–364, 1994

Woods JH, Katz JL, Winger G: Benzodiazepines: use, abuse and consequences. Pharmacol Rev 44:151–347, 1992

Woody SR, Sanderson, WC: Manuals for empirically supported treatments: 1998 update from the task force on psychological interventions. Clin Psychol 51:17–21, 1998

Appendix: Internet Resources

American Psychiatric Association
  http://www.psych.org

American Psychological Association
  http://www.apa.org

Anxiety Disorders Association of America
  http://www.adaa.org

Association for the Advancement of Behavior Therapy
  http://www.aabt.org

National Alliance for the Mentally Ill
  http://www.nami.org

National Institute of Mental Health
  http://www.nimh.nih.gov
  Anxiety disorders: http://www.nimh.nih.gov/anxiety

National Library of Medicine
  http://www.nlm.nih.gov/

Obsessive-Compulsive Foundation
  http://www.ocfoundation.org

The Panic Center
  http://www.paniccenter.net

Trichotillomania Learning Center
  http://www.trich.org

Index

Page numbers printed in **boldface** *type refer to tables or figures.*

175